HELP! I AM SURROUNDED

~ BY ~

BITCHES

HELP! I AM SURROUNDED

~ BY ~

BITCHES

THE SWAMP GODDESS GUIDE TO FRIENDSHIP FRENZY
AMID MENOPAUSAL MAYHEM AND AGING ANGST

Wendy Kyman, Ph.D

Help! I Am Surrounded By Bitches:
The Swamp Goddess Guide to Friendship Frenzy Amid
Menopausal Mayhem and Aging Angst

First Edition 2013
Copyright © 2013 Wendy Kyman, Ph.D.
All Rights Reserved.

Published by: Wiloworks
www.wiloworks.com

Book Cover and Design by Jesse Scaturro, www.jessescaturro.com

Printed in United States of America

Library of Congress Control Number 2012932396

ISBN: 09882795-0-9

Note To Readers: This book is intended to provide opinions and ideas. The author and publisher are not rendering professional services to individual readers. The suggestions in this book are not to be used for psychological advice, diagnosis or treatment. Nor are they intended t o substitute for actual psychological counseling.

Dedicated to my mom and first friend – Tess Kyman

She would have loved the title

And to beloved aunt Helen Starman

CONTENTS

CHAPTER 1

DOUBLE MILESTONE CHANGES

What a twisted cosmic joke. Nearly all women get caught in the grip of menopause just as we hit our 50th birthdays. Two potent milestones swoop into our lives almost at once.

This double milestone often triggers profound life changes as women review our past and envision the future. It is not possible to distinguish whether menopause or turning 50 (to many, the official stamp of midlife) is the specific catalyst. Nor does the precise cause really matter. For now, let's agree that two milestones equal twice the potential for change.

At this pivotal time, women turn inward; a change we welcome. Double milestoners pay particular attention to what is relevant to us, such as

✪ We notice variations in our temperament, patience, and tolerance levels.

Do you know any temperamental, impatient, intolerant women?

☻ We get furious when our feelings, thoughts, and opinions are ignored or dismissed.
Doesn't that seem to be happening a lot lately?

☻ We are not in the mood for thoughtless, rude, unkind individuals.
Don't they seem to be everywhere?

☻ We seem to regard fewer and fewer people and places as sources of comfort.
Have you been craving *alone time*?

Then, to the utter amazement of us all, double milestoners realize it is not just anonymous persons, but supposedly close friends who are the source of our discomfort, resentment, and anger? Or, women are informed it is *we* who are the source of a friend's discomfort, resentment, and anger. Impossible!

FOOD FOR THOUGHT

Given that our friends are experiencing their own version of menopausal mayhem and aging angst, it's not only possible, but also probable. Gasp!

It's no wonder women are caught off-guard when encountering double milestone friendship frenzy. It has been virtually unacknowledged and undisclosed, until now, that some longstanding friendships spontaneously combust, while others seem to be on a low simmer during this season of women's lives.

Effective ways to shed light on friendship frenzy include acknowledging and disclosing the questions we regularly ask ourselves.

Here are a few.

☸ Is it me? Am I the only one who is often confused, frequently amazed, and increasingly annoyed at most things my friends say and do?

☸ Is it me? Have I been doing something that turns the women I thought were friends into shrieking, nagging, whining, self-centered shrews?

☸ Is it me? Were my friends like this all along and it's only now I am noticing what I previously ignored?

☸ Is it me? If I met these women today, would I choose them as friends? Would they choose me?

☸ Is it me? Are there others chanting the silent roar, 'Help! I am surrounded by bitches' – oops, I mean friends.

FOOD FOR THOUGHT

Keep in mind, everything is a bit over the top during menopausal mayhem and aging angst.

Join The Swamp Goddess journey to
☸ ease your passage through the murky waters of menopausal/aging friendships

- establish friendship criteria

- choose which friends to keep, those to let go, and know the difference

- create quality friendships

We all know the goddess thing is somewhat overdone. So what? Swamp Goddesses do not care about such things.

FOOD FOR THOUGHT

The documented average age of menopause is 51. There is no precise documented age for the onset of midlife. According to conventional thought and opinion, midlife begins in earnest at 50. However, your milestone moment may arrive at 43, 65, 92, or any age in between.

HELPFUL HINT

Midlife is usually the stage of life most of us begin to acknowledge we are aging. Thus, 'midlife' and 'aging' are used interchangeably in *Help! I Am Surrounded By Bitches: The Swamp Goddess Guide To Friendship Frenzy Amid Menopausal Mayhem And Aging Angst.*

CHAPTER 2

BIRTH OF SWAMP GODDESS

How did I evolve from an uncomfortable, cranky, 50ish, menopausal woman suffering from hideous hot flashes, drenching night sweats, and interrupted sleep (plus other dreadful signs and symptoms) to Swamp Goddess?

MY STORY

I am a college professor. Teaching is a bit like performing. I have to *entertain* a classroom full of bright young adults, hold their attention for extended stretches, present new material in a coherent, intelligent manner, and be sufficiently alert to correctly respond to unfathomable queries. Obviously, concentration and focus are required.

Sleep disturbances interfere with my professional life and do serious damage to my appearance. Does anyone find the red, swollen, baggy-eyed look attractive? No, I don't think so.

One typical menopausal night, I woke up for the zillionth time. I was lying in my soggy bed, soaking wet with perspiration. Maybe I should be ladylike and pretend I was glistening and glowing in a dewy sort of way. Spare me.

When I awaken like this, I go through my usual routine. I check the clock, find out if I slept more than 45 minutes, determine how many hours I have left before the alarm clock rings, take a drink of water, double check the air conditioner is running, triple check the large stand-up fan is blowing cool air on me, wipe up gobs of sweat (er…uh…beads of dew), and struggle to fall back to sleep.

On this special night, something life-changing happened. When I woke up at 3 AM, I was immersed in a transcendent experience. I was not in my bed, in my bedroom, or even in my apartment. Somehow, I had been mysteriously transported to a swamp. There could be no other explanation for how my body and bedding were so waterlogged.

Swamps are filled with water. Swamp dwellers are perpetually wet. Swamp dwellers cannot rely on luxuriously high thread-count sheets, swirling fans, or monster air conditioners. Not one of those items has the ability to overpower the elements of a swamp. In other words, when you are in a swamp, you *are* in a swamp.

The image of the swamp took hold rather quickly. It perfectly depicted what I was experiencing each and every night for the past forever. And just like that, I embraced the absurd notion of swamp living. Next, it seemed fitting to anoint myself goddess of my swamp. Hooray! Swamp Goddess was born.

I visualized myself as Botticelli's Birth of Venus. Do you know the painting of a woman standing in water on a half shell? Because it was my visualization, as an added bonus, I took the liberty of imagining myself looking just as fabulous as she. Why not?

I did think of other identities. I could have called myself Damp Diva, Moist Mama, Hothouse Hannah, or Hortense the Hottie. I liked those but, for me, the name Swamp Goddess was perfect. I still love it.

As I settled into my newly created swamp universe, I released the anxiety concerning my ability to function the following day with only three hours of sleep. Rather than calculating the hours left before I had to be up and about, I contemplated a fresh approach to menopause and aging.

A fresh approach must include adjusting my double milestone perspective. Admittedly, previous to this special night, I had focused on the gloomy, ominous information presented in the vast array of menopause and aging related books, articles, and research I usually read. Surely this negativity was not helpful.

Depending on the day, I labeled my state of being as 'hormonal meltdown,' 'perpetual PMS,' 'ditz on display,' or the pitiful classic, 'absent minded professor.' I was obsessed with estimating when the menopausal/aging wretchedness would vanish so I could get back to my old (younger) self.

Enough. I was done.

Unexpectedly, I began to laugh, really laugh. I laughed at the insidious way double milestone woes catapulted into my life and brought about my current circumstance. Have I actually embraced living in a swamp? As I was enjoying this zany interlude, my laughter instigated a reality check – menopausal misery and aging angst may last awhile. Yikes!

Questions started swirling.

- Do I have to live in a swamp five weeks, five months, five years, forever?

- Will the absurdity get worse before it gets better?

- What am I going to do?

What I had to do was come up with a feasible, durable, and potentially lifelong plan to cope with double milestone signs and symptoms. Whatever the plan, I needed supplies – primarily, massive amounts of energy. At this point, I was not sure I had any in reserve.

My thoughts wandered off on a hazy, insomnia-induced tangent regarding sources of energy.

I pondered.

- Do we each have a personal *power plant* producing abundant amounts of energy?

- Is it possible to generate enough supplies to fill our seemingly bottomless double milestone needs?

I wondered.

❂ Are double milestoners appreciative and protective of our energy supplies?

❂ Do we recklessly (unintentionally) give away our supplies? To whom?

❂ How can we safeguard ourselves from those who routinely devour our energy?

For those of us in one-sided relationships who generously give away enormous amounts of unreciprocated energy – say it out loud, ' No More!' As women enduring menopausal misery and aging angst, we must conserve what we have in order to fuel us through.

FOOD FOR THOUGHT

Reciprocal relationships enjoy a healthy exchange of resources. We recharge each other. One-sided relationships are unhealthy. We are drained of our energy because we get virtually nothing in return.

Conservation plans ushered in a wave of optimism. I looked forward to the profound shift that would come once I implemented the overall strategy to be goddess of my swamp and conservator of my energy supplies. What wonderful symbolism for truly owning my life.

Hold On. It all sounded fantastic, but I had to get practical.

❂ What does *owning my life* actually mean in the real

world, in my world?

✪ How do I function day-to-day as Swamp Goddess?

Searching for answers, again I got sidetracked (another double milestone *gift*) and began floating in and out of layer upon layer of uninvited flashbacks.

At this point in life, along with hot flashes and distractions, double milestoners get recurrent flashbacks. Folks in our age group reflect on where we have been, what we have done, and who has accompanied us along the way. We tend to critique past choices, roads taken and not taken, also blessings and regrets.

Perhaps coincidentally, perhaps not, previous to my birth as Swamp Goddess, I had been preoccupied with reviewing my life. It did not take much creativity to label this The Midlife Review.

My Midlife Review was filled with 'would haves,' 'should haves,' 'could haves.' Ordinarily, whenever I reflected on my 'wouldas, shouldas, couldas,' and faced my regrets, I was comforted by the hope I still was able to make meaningful changes to my life.

FOOD FOR THOUGHT

As you know, approaching life with a positive attitude is extraordinarily beneficial. A good plan is to assume we double milestoners have ample time ahead and proceed to live life to the fullest.

Recently, The Midlife Review has led to thoughts of The End of Life Review. Ideally, this is a long way into the future. Nevertheless, I wonder what it will reveal. I certainly do not want any 'wouldas, shouldas, couldas' haunting me at the end of my life. May I assume you share the same ambition?

As soon as I surfaced from my meandering flashbacks and resumed my Swamp Goddess musings, I amended my goals for The End of Life Review. It was essential to incorporate my brand new revelations. The revised objectives for my End of Life Review had to reflect life lived as Swamp Goddess.

As this remarkable and transformative night ended, I solidified The Swamp Goddess Lifestyle Basics.

Swamp Goddesses

❂ own our lives

❂ safeguard our energy supplies

❂ have a no-regrets policy

To accomplish our goals, we

❂ choose what we want

❂ let go of what we don't

and

❂ know the difference

The birth of Swamp Goddess was powerful. I sense this experience was not random for me, nor will it be for you. Swamp Goddess is born at exactly the right moment to ensure we do what is necessary to own our lives.

FOOD FOR THOUGHT

What are the prevalent themes of your Midlife Review?

Is one specific past situation or relationship the focal point of your 'wouldas, shouldas, couldas?'

Do you have goals for your End of Life Review?

NOTE

Are you thinking you're not qualified to be Swamp Goddess because you do not get hot flashes or night sweats? Nonsense! Of course you are cordially invited to be Swamp Goddess. Consider yourself lucky. You managed to inhabit a dry patch of the swamp. I am sure your menopausal mayhem and aging angst manifest in other ways.

CHAPTER 3

THE SWAMP GODDESS LIFESTYLE

For double milestoners (and others), The Swamp Goddess persona symbolizes owning our lives, safeguarding our energy supplies, and living with a no-regrets policy. We choose what we want, let go of what we don't, and know the difference.

As your wise, thoughtful minds evaluate the proposal to adopt The Swamp Goddess lifestyle, I expect a number of responses.

☻ A group of you are thinking, 'Swamp Goddess sounds intriguing in a warm, fuzzy, and slightly goofy sort of way. What the heck, I'll try it out.' Great. Get ready for an adventure.

☻ Others are swayed by the idea of taking a close look at double milestone friendships. I know you feel something is brewing, or just plain out of whack, with your friends. I am glad to go through this process with you.

☿ Some of you are exclaiming, 'been there, done that.' You're already living life as the goddess you are. Good. You have the basics. Then again, you have not reaped the benefits of The Swamp Goddess Friendship Assessment. Your goddess self will be enhanced.

☿ Undoubtedly, there are those who are resistant to the whole goddess thing. You may be saying, 'who do I think I am calling myself a goddess?' C'mon. Give embracing your goddess self a chance.

☿ Or are you thinking, 'hasn't the goddess, diva thing been overdone?' No. And furthermore, Swamp Goddesses do not care about such things.

I have added a dose of humor to The Swamp Goddess world. We are all aware it is irrational to feel anything is humorous when we are sleep deprived, uncomfortable, and irritable. Nothing else has worked. Why not give this a try? Center your tongue firmly in your cheek and enter The Swamp Goddess world. We welcome you.

Despite the attempts at humor, there is fierce acknowledgement this is a difficult and, for some of us, awful time in our lives. Let's be blunt. Menopause sucks; aging is humbling.

As a health educator, I eat healthy foods, exercise regularly, blah, blah blah. I get irate when women are given advice, such as, 'modifying eating habits, increasing exercise, reducing stress levels, and more blah, blah will diminish menopausal and midlife related signs.' I wish.

Aren't you annoyed by the platitudes, 'age is just a number,' 'you are as old as you feel,' or the recent, '60 is the new 40.' More wishes.

Have you tried various remedies for your personal brand of menopausal misery and aging angst? I have. Most double milestoners have. If we miraculously do find a bit of relief, it is usually temporary and we revert to status-quo with at least a couple, but probably more, nasty symptoms.

We continue to have vicious hot flashes, night sweats, interrupted sleep, foggy brain, memory lapses, unanticipated aches and pains, emotional meltdowns, and more.

Yet, here I am encouraging you to try another approach, The Swamp Goddess lifestyle. It comes highly recommended.

Next, you may be asking, 'Why do double milestoners need to adopt The Swamp Goddess lifestyle now?' The reply is simple. 'If not now, when?' We are already undergoing changes. It is sensible to use these changes to enrich our lives.

As we stagger through menopausal mayhem and aging angst, our relationships are becoming noticeably unsettled. Many of our connections with romantic partners, family, friends, and colleagues are shifting. Some are strained; others are shaky. Several have already disintegrated. Happily, a precious few relationships are strong (ummmm …

depending on the day).

For now, we narrow our focus to friendships. Needless to say, we do not snap our fingers, immediately transform into Swamp Goddesses, and have blissful, quality friendships. If I had a magic wand and could make that possible, I would merrily wave it nonstop.

Patience is not my best attribute. Nonetheless, the Swamp Goddess lifestyle of choosing the friends we want, letting go of those we don't, and knowing the difference – all with no regrets – is worth the time and effort.

How do double milestoners get from *here* to *there*?

We begin by viewing our friends through a specially designed lens, The Swamp Goddess Friendship Assessment.

CHAPTER 4

THE SWAMP GODDESS FRIENDSHIP ASSESSMENT (SGFA)

PORTION 1 – INTRODUCTION

OBJECTIVE

To choose which friends to keep, those to let go, and know the difference.

DESCRIPTION

The Swamp Goddess Friendship Assessment (SGFA) is an opportunity to view friendships using The Swamp Goddess Lens.

You will develop the ability to choose which friends to keep, those to let go, and know the difference. Do not worry about letting go. I will help by providing clear-cut strategies and useful solutions. We must remove what we don't want in order to let in what we do want. It's quite refreshing to say goodbye to a few (or many) expired friendships.

As an added benefit, you'll acquire skills to create quality friendships that fit perfectly into The Swamp Goddess lifestyle.

FOOD FOR THOUGHT

The SGFA requires time and concentration. Many of us are short on both. To ease the situation, pick your preferred timetable. Either complete the entire SGFA all at once, or do some now, and the rest later.

SGFA Portion 2 is waiting for you in The Appendix section. Get to it after you complete Portion 1, finish reading Help! I Am Surrounded By Bitches…, or whenever you are ready.

HELPFUL HINTS

As with everything else in life, the more thought and attention you give The Swamp Goddess Friendship Assessment, the more you will get out of it. There will be a return on your investment.

I strongly urge completing The Swamp Goddess Friendship Assessment Portions 1 & 2. It is worth your while to do both. You are worth your while.

CHAPTER 5

THE SWAMP GODDESS FRIENDSHIP ASSESSMENT (SGFA)

PART A – MAKING A LIST – CHECKING IT TWICE

OBJECTIVE
To identify friends

DIRECTIONS
Use paper and pen to record your responses.

❂ Conjure up the faces of current and past friends. See them as if you are skimming through a photo album.

❂ Monitor the emotions evoked by these images.

❂ It is fine to focus more on some friends and less on others.

❂ Make a list of all the faces you have pictured.

⊛ When that preliminary list is complete, check your phone book, email directories, and holiday card addresses for the friends you have omitted. Don't forget social media sites.

⊛ Add these additional names to your list.

⊛ Your completed friends' list may be extremely short or very long.

⊛ If you want to organize your list, try creating categories, such as close and distant friends, current and past friends, business and neighbor friends, or another designation that suits you.

FOOD FOR THOUGHT

As the process unfolds, you will see patterns overlap all categories of friendships.

HELPFUL HINTS

You need a notepad and pen.

Make at least 10 copies of your list.

CHAPTER 6

THE SWAMP GODDESS FRIENDSHIP ASSESSMENT (SGFA)

PART B – HELP! I AM SURROUNDED BY BITCHES

OBJECTIVE
To identify personalities of friends

DESCRIPTION
The undesirable personality types depicted in this portion of The Swamp Goddess Friendship Assessment are personified using a notorious cast of characters. Each character is housed into a Family.

You will note, within each Family, there are similarities among members – as is typical in any family. Some Family members, and their corresponding traits, are more closely related than others. They may be sisters, cousins, or distant aunts.

The characters and their stories are composite sketches amassed during my 25+ years working with countless women from diverse backgrounds. Names and unique identifiers are disguised to protect confidentiality. When applicable, I have included my personal stories.

DIRECTIONS
Use paper and pen to record your responses.

☺ If you did not make a friends' list, do so now. You will gain more from this section if your friends' names are written down. (Chapter 5 has instructions.)

☺ Read all Family descriptions.

☺ As you make your way through the descriptions below, look for Families and personality types that resemble each friend on your list.

☺ When you match a Family member and a friend, write the Family's name next the friend's name.

HELPFUL HINTS

Here are some probable results.

☺ The same Family member will be placed next to most, maybe all, of your friends. Notice a trend?

☺ A few friends will have more than one Family member placed next to them.

☺ Certain Family member descriptions will precisely fit your friends; others will not. Feel free to tweak, add, or subtract characteristics to exactly match each friend.

THE FAMILIES

Recognize anyone?

1 THE OPERA SINGER FAMILY

Members of this Family are extraordinarily self-absorbed. When first meeting them, we assume they are singing scales I, I, I, ME, ME, ME …

Opera Singers are rampant. They inhabit most big cities, small towns, and local neighborhoods. It is reasonable to assume you know more than one member of The Opera Singer Family.

IMPORTANT IDA

Important Ida is the matriarch of The Opera Singer Family. From her self-absorbed perspective, Ida's needs, concerns, and interests are so important they take precedence before anyone and everyone. It rarely enters Ida's egocentric mind that others have needs, concerns, and interests – especially if they do not duplicate hers.

FOOD FOR THOUGHT

Respect, consideration, thoughtfulness, and reciprocity are key ingredients in Swamp Goddess friendships. No matter if searching here, there, and everywhere, these traits will never be found in relationships with Important Ida. Never.

PATTY'S STORY

Have you had an experience comparable to Patty's 50th Big Birthday story?

Charlotte and Patty became friends when they both lived in North Carolina. Their friendship continued despite Charlotte's relocation to Arizona. For months prior to Charlotte's Big Birthday, she frequently called Patty. Charlotte began her calls by weeping in dread of turning 50. Patty indulged her friend with soothing charm and lighthearted humor.

Charlotte pleaded with Patty to travel to Arizona for her birthday. Charlotte was convinced turning 50 was an event she could not face without Patty.

Consider this: Charlotte would not be alone on her 50th. She lived with her husband and two sons. Moreover, she had several friends in Arizona ready to celebrate. On the other hand, Patty was hesitant to leave her elderly mother. And, she despised traveling anywhere by plane.

Although Patty was aware of Charlotte's Important Ida leanings, in the spirit of friendship, she put aside her reluctance and unease. Patty went to Arizona.

You know the story does not end there. Less than one year later, it was Patty's 50th. Unexpectedly, she was feeling a bit of the same dread Charlotte had described just months before.

Patty wanted Charlotte's companionship to get through The Big Birthday blues. By the way, Patty was single and her children were away at college.

But, Charlotte's need had passed. She stopped her frequent calls. When Patty asked for comfort, do you think Charlotte reciprocated Patty's generosity? Did Charlotte make herself available? Was she traveling to North Carolina and spending Patty's 50th with her? No, no, and no.

Charlotte's status as Important Ida was confirmed. She dismissed Patty's feelings by saying, '50 is no biggie.' Charlotte had her birthday and was over it; therefore Patty should get over it.

Because she is a typical Important Ida, Charlotte truly believed saying, 'no biggie' had magical powers and Patty's feelings related to turning 50 would (and should) instantly vanish. Poof! All gone.

FRIENDSHIP STATUS
Patty no longer responds to Charlotte's one-sided friendship.

ONE-WAY JUANITA

Juanita and Ida are Opera Singer sisters. Although their *all about me* personality traits are similar, if you look closely you can spot subtle differences in the sisters' behaviors.

Juanita is more adept than Ida in covering her disregard for others' needs, concerns, and thoughts. From time-to-time, Juanita surprises her friends by making an *effort* to give compelling reasons (excuses) explaining why we cannot count on her.

Friends have to guard against being duped by Juanita's finely-tuned skills. Be especially wary of befriending a Juanita who is so skilled, she tricks herself into believing her own bogus justifications.

FOOD FOR THOUGHT

In quality friendships, we count on each other.

MY STORY #1

I had a long-distance friendship. When both of us were younger, we regularly visited each other. With the passing years, busy lives intervened and our friendship dwindled to phone calls.

Relying solely on calls, without the usual distraction of other people and activities, it became glaringly obvious my friend was a One-Way Juanita. She talked endlessly about herself – her life, work, activities, family – on and on and on. After Juanita finished imparting her *important* news, she would exclaim, 'I am so exhausted by *our* conversation. I have to hang up.' Seriously.

When I first became consciously aware of the one-sided nature of the chats, I was stunned. What promted me to finally notice my friend's behavior? How had I accepted this treatment from a friend? Has the relationship always been one-sided?

Evidently, in pre-Swamp Goddess days, I was a sap for Juanitas and did not diligently safeguard my energy supplies. I recklessly squandered resources on innumerable Juanita characters. Being Swamp Goddess enabled me to gain an awareness of Opera Singer personalities, particularly Juanitas, and my tendency to give away too much of myself to them.

Before I had a chance to formulate a plan to address Juanita's no longer acceptable actions, she called with a problem and asked for advice. I gave her whatever help I could and told myself it was not the appropriate time to discuss her Juanita ways. Maybe, I just did not feel ready for the necessary discussion.

When we finished straightening out her dilemma, she said, 'If you want to talk about what is going on with you, call me back so you can pay the long-distance cost for your side of the conversation.' (Prior to cell phones, fees were charged for long-distance calls.)

You cannot make up anything this ghastly, nor can you be

prepared for it. I was so flustered by my friend's statement, it stands out as one of the few times in my life I was totally speechless. To add irony to the story, this Juanita judges communication as the primary ingredient of good relationships. How bizarre.

FRIENDSHIP STATUS

My ability to speak recovered, but the friendship did not. I was done accommodating this woman's One-Way Juanita behavior. For a while, my soon-to-be ex friend tried to coax back the 'old' me. As an authentic Opera Singer, she would not, or could not, change her ways. The relationship was doomed.

MY STORY #2

I moved from an apartment where I had lived for 20 years. The moving process took place during the college semester while I was busy teaching, counseling, as well as, attending to my other work related and life activities.

I hired large, burly men and a big truck for the actual move, but I was on my own to sort through, and pack up, my belongings. Concurrently, I had to get my new apartment livable. Everything needed to be done within a few weeks.

All of us, at least once, have gone through this arduous process. Everyone knows how physically and emotionally exhausting it is. Whatever assistance anyone gives is welcome. Gratefully, a friend volunteered to lend a hand. I eagerly accepted. Keep in mind, I never asked. She offered.

This was another Juanita friend; I had quite a few. She repeatedly broke dates, but continually promised to lend that hand. My friend did finally show up … one month *later* when I was already settled into my new home.

My friend's Juanita ways were flagrantly displayed.

⚙ Was Juanita embarrassed? No

⚙ Did I remain friends with her? Yes

⚙ Does the story continue? Absolutely

Almost two years later, this Juanita also moved. She actually asked me to spend an entire weekend helping pack up her house. The request is made even more spectacular because Juanita's husband and three teenagers were available to share the workload. Okay, maybe not share, but available to do something.

What is it with Opera Singers? Was my friend using and abusing my tendency to let her zap my energy? Or, did she get selective amnesia? Is it really possible this Juanita forgot what she did *not* do for me less than two years earlier when I moved without her promised assistance? I am thrilled to report, I remembered.

Another possibility: Juanita was being true to her personality. She convinced herself that her excuses for not being there for my move were valid. I know. It is The Opera Singer performing her solo. Can you hear it – I, I, I, Me, Me, Me.

FRIENDSHIP STATUS
I had crossed the threshold and was fully Swamp Goddess

by the time of *this* incident with *this* One-Way Juanita. My response was a simple, 'I can't.' The audacity of her request did not warrant any discussion, justification, or explanation. I bet you agree.

The experience was both painful and joyful. For Juanita to shamelessly ask my assistance with her move, despite her disregard for mine, took my breath away.

I ached with pain for my pre-Swamp Goddess self who never challenged her or any of my other Juanita friends. By not doing so, I allowed Juanitas to regard their one-way behaviors as acceptable.

Ultimately, I take responsibility for not protecting myself. Never again. My Swamp Goddess gear is fully lined with anti-Opera Singer shields.

This Juanita's actions also gave me tremendous joy. I exalted in the stark difference between before and after The Swamp Goddess persona. The ease with which I was able to say 'no' was extremely gratifying. Without hesitation or doubt, I was adamant in knowing I was done with each and every one of my One-Way Juanita friends.

MY STATUS

I vow to never again squander energy supplies on unappreciative, self-absorbed Opera Singers. Yay!

I vow to focus on reciprocal relationships filled with respect, kindness, consideration, thoughtfulness, and reciprocity. One-Way Juanitas need not apply. Double Yay!!

VICTORIA THE VERBAL VOMITER aka VVV
Victoria's status in The Opera Singer Family is legendary. She is easy to recognize. VVV is so busy babbling nonstop about *her* favorite topic, *herself, her* mouth is in perpetual motion.

In Victoria's world, conversations are monologues – *hers.* Anyone in VVV's presence is there merely to serve as *her* audience.

FOOD FOR THOUGHT

When describing an Opera Singer, note the frequent use of 'her.' It truly is all about her.

There are two typical scenarios with Victoria: in-person meetings and phone conversations.

In-Person With VVV
A group of holdouts go with Victoria for dinner and drinks. These friends continue holding out hope Victoria will change. They believe this time will be different and are looking forward to an evening of juicy girl-talk. The women are either ridiculously optimistic or downright delusional.

Even before appetizers are served, a VVV reality-check hits the friends upside the head. Victoria does not, will not, and probably cannot, hush up. As usual, it is a battle for any of her companions to get in a word or two.

Oh, here it is. At some point there seems to be an opening

when VVV takes a sip of wine or a bite of food. One enthu-siastic woman thinks, 'Ahhh, finally my turn.'

Not so fast. If someone other than VVV chimes in using the word 'I,' Victoria's eyes glaze over. She gets fidgety and twitchy as she looks around the room, at her watch, in her purse, any-where but at the speaker. Frequently, Victoria chooses that moment to use the bathroom or make an urgent call.

When the group steers the conversation back toward VVV, she stops squirming and returns to her endless run-on sentences.

Phone Calls With VVV
Some of us are unwilling to spend time with Victoria. Fur-thermore, we do not call her. Most double milestoners don't have the patience for endless one-sided babble.

As you know, there are holdouts still taking VVV's calls. Why? A typical phone call with VVV goes something like this. The phone rings. We answer it with 'hello.' Normal enough. It is Victoria on the phone. Do not expect normal.

VVV whispers a perfunctory 'hi.' She immediately launches into her vomiting routine. Words just spill forth. She never asks if we are busy, on our way out the door, rushing to an appointment, or … possibly, maybe, perhaps … making love.

Nothing her friends are doing matters when Victoria needs to vomit. In some cases, Victoria does not care who answers the phone. Her concern is to have a receptacle for – you know what. Ick!

Similar to the in-person scenario with VVV, at precisely the moment her friend dares interject a sentence beginning with 'I,' Victoria pretends something has just come up and must end the *conversation.*

If Victoria does stay on for her friend's turn, VVV's lack of attention echoes through the phone lines. She can be heard typing on the computer, talking to her dog, changing television channels, anything but actually listening.

Are we receiving Victoria's message? She is not interested in what others have to say. In VVV's distorted version of listening, the act of cradling the phone and not hanging up is her twisted concept of friendship.

Making an Effort VVV style

Victoria thinks her friendship responsibility is to sporadically make a VVV type effort during a friend's side the conversation. For these special events, she mumbles noises as an alternative to her usual dead silence. VVV's responses reflect her disinterest – a combination of 'uh huhs,' 'mmmms,' and 'ohs.'

There are rare occasions when Victoria rewards her friends with a trite statement. She actually imagines others are tricked into believing this offering, pawned off as wisdom, is useful. Aren't we so over her already?

I know of one VVV who should have trademarked the phrase, 'this too shall pass.' It is her go-to response when she is *fake listening.* This VVV is convinced these empty words (when used as a one-phrase-fits-all) are enough to end her friend's side of the conversation.

This Victoria states, 'this too shall pass' so often, it has become a joke among the people in her life. She has no clue. Then again, why are people still in her life? No clue.

Senior VVVs

Have you come in contact with VVVs who use the *senior moment* excuse for interrupting when someone else is speaking? They claim, 'I do not mean to interrupt (so don't), but if I do not say this now, I will forget.' What is your reaction?

These senior VVVs are telling us their rudeness is justified because what they have to announce is of more interest and importance than whatever topic we are discussing. This gets my blood boiling. I usually reply by mentioning I have senior moments as well and continue with what I was saying. Sometimes it works, sometimes it doesn't.

FOOD FOR THOUGHT

Swamp Goddesses refuse to sit silently through an encounter with Verbal Vomiters and, most certainly, reject even the imagery of being receptacles. Swamp Goddesses love to have conversations with our friends. We know ideal communication consists of dialogues. Each person contributes by speaking, listening, and sharing information. Listening is essential. At no time – past, present, or future – will Verbal Vomiters have the ability, or the desire, to listen and engage in dialogues.

How is it possible for VVVs to have friends willing to endure their behavior? Here are three possibilities.

1. Each gets her needs met.

For any number of reasons, some people are taciturn. They do not want to share personal thoughts, feelings, and information. Thus, the privacy needs of uncommunicative folks are met by VVVs.

2. VVVs pounce on the courteous and well mannered.

Many double milestoners were raised to believe it is good manners to listen when others are speaking and to subdue the need to be the center of attention. Women with these notions of polite behavior must beware of pouncing VVVs.

3. Disturbing cases of erroneous messaging.

A few take the polite behavior notions to disturbing levels. They scold themselves with rebukes such as, 'I am boring, selfish, and rude,' when wanting a turn to vocalize thoughts and feelings. These misguided individuals worry that talking about themselves places too much 'burden' on their friends.

Frankly, they communicate the message, 'my news is not important because I am not important.' Or to put it bluntly, 'my role in this conversation is to be the container for VVV's vomit.' Yuck!

To add more bluntness, being someone's receptacle is not friendship, and it certainly is not polite.

THE TWINS
CONNIE THE CONTESTANT AND
OLIVIA THE OLYMPIAN

Connie and Olivia are The Opera Singer Family twins. These two are always competing with their friends, relentlessly aiming to accumulate Gold Medals. The twins win when their needs and concerns are judged the most important and garner all the attention.

If we go through a difficult situation, the twins declare their situation is worse. If a friend has a headache, the twins *see* the headache and *raise* with a migraine. If our son wins an award, their son wins two awards. You get the picture.

FOOD FOR THOUGHT

Connie and Olivia not only dismiss their friends' concerns as frivolous, but they use our personal stories as jumping off points to recite their supposed more serious needs. The twins expect us to forget our concerns, problems, and needs in order to focus on them. For Opera Singers it is always I, I, I, Me, Me, Me.

ROSALIE'S STORY

Rosalie loved tennis. Twice a week she played doubles as part of a foursome. After a vigorous game, Rosalie and two of her companions left the competition at the courts. The women wanted tranquil lunches and relaxed conversation.

The fourth member of the group, JoAnne, refused to give up the competition. During lunch, JoAnne turned the women's discussions into quests for Gold. She kept pushing until she felt her stories *won.*

Within a short time, the three double milestone tennis players grew irritated with JoAnne. They narrowed the choices: oust JoAnne from their tennis game, exclude her from post-game lunches, or directly address the issue.

The women chose the latter option. They told JoAnne her competitive streak was welcome on the tennis court, but to 'give it a rest' when they were off the court – or she no longer would be welcome to share lunches.

FRIENDSHIP STATUS

JoAnne respected her friends' forthrightness. She took what the three women presented as a challenge. From then on, whenever the tennis players went to lunch, JoAnne paid the entire bill if she behaved like Connie the Contestant or Olivia the Olympian. In this way, she continued competing – with herself.

ACCOMMODATE ME AMY

As a member of The Opera Singer Family, Amy is a cousin to Juanita and Ida. Amy alleges she is very, very busy doing very, very important … who cares. We are not impressed.

Amy's friends must adhere to her schedule. It dictates when she and her friends get together. She is free Wednesday for a 6:30AM breakfast. If such an early time does not meet our timetable, Amy persists until she gets her way.

Amy puts pressure on her friends. She relentlessly asks questions, such as, 'you can't make it? Does this mean you do not want to spend time together? What exactly are your plans for Wednesday at 6:30AM?'

Amy expects friends to tell her their daily tasks and appointments so she can determine whether previously planned activities can be rearranged. We find ourselves appeasing Amy to avoid the hassle or the explanation. This is how Amy gets her way – until her friends finally and firmly refuse to give in.

Design a suitable strategy if your Accommodate Me Amy is nagging you to spend time together that fits her schedule – not yours, and to do things she wants – with no concern for your preferences.

Agree to meet with your Annie friend and take the lead. Do not do what she wants, when she wants, and where she wants. Go to an event you choose and have dinner at your favorite restaurant.

If you need to tackle chores, take Annie with you. See if she sticks around as you do laundry, feed the dog, and go grocery shopping.

FOOD FOR THOUGHT

Be prepared. Your Accommodate Me Annie friend may choose to end the friendship because you no longer serve her Opera Singer needs. Bye, Bye.

MORE FOOD FOR THOUGHT

Most members of The Opera Singer Family will never expand their consciousness to grasp someone else's reality. Swamp Goddesses do not fool ourselves into thinking we can transform their self-centered ways. It helps to know, really know, all we can transform is our reaction to Opera Singers' demands. It is acceptable, permissible, and downright obligatory to say, 'NO.'

REMINDER

No justifications and no explanations are necessary.

DORIS'S STORY

Doris's menopausal insomnia keeps her awake until the wee hours of the morning. She has announced her sleeping woes to anyone within earshot, including her friend Penny.

On the flip side, Penny contends she suffers no menopausal sleep disturbances and continues her lifelong routine of rising early. She incessantly presses Doris to meet for 7AM breakfasts, refusing to accept that morning meetings are not doable for Doris. As a member of The Opera Singer Family, Penny cannot envision anyone having a sleep schedule that differs from hers.

Doris has come up with a tactic to offset her friend's Accommodate Me Annie pushiness. Because Doris is awake late at night, she suggests midnight as a counter-offer to 7AM. Penny laughs this off as a ridiculous joke. (She is in bed by 9PM.) Doris hopes Penny will eventually get the message that a midnight rendezvous for Penny is comparable to a 7AM one for Doris.

FRIENDSHIP STATUS

Currently, Penny and Doris meet for afternoon outings that suit both their schedules. Simple.

ELAINE'S STORY

Elaine works from home. When she has a heavy workload with deadlines to meet, Elaine informs her friends she is unavailable. Her Opera Singer friend Kate stubbornly refuses to accept the concept of people doing *real* work from their homes. After all, Kate works in an office and has set hours. Surely, Elaine is free to take extended breaks from her 'make believe' work – to focus on Kate.

Elaine devised a way to get her friend Kate to respect her

working conditions. On one of Elaine's workdays, she agreed when Kate invited herself to come for a visit. Elaine spent the day working. Kate spent the day watching Elaine work – until Kate got bored and walked out.

FRIENDSHIP STATUS

Elaine is persistent and continues devising innovative ways to convince her friend that life does not revolve around Kate. Good luck doing that with an Opera Singer.

THE TRIPLETS
OPPORTUNISTIC OPAL, MOOCHING MINIE,
and YOLANDA THE USER

Look out for these Opera Singer Triplets. Their names say it all.

Let's begin with Opal. She views everyone, including friends, as opportunities to exploit. To help avoid being suckered in by Opal's cunning ways, friends need a constant reminder of her personality. A good idea is to imagine Opal's forehead tattooed with the motto 'what can you do for me?'

FOOD FOR THOUGHT

Swamp Goddesses are generous and kind. Some individuals mistake our kindness for weakness and think we are suckers. This is a big error. We are generous and kind, but we are not fools.

MORE FOOD FOR THOUGHT

Self-preservation is noble and wise.

SANDRA'S STORY

At age 48, Sandra returned to school for her Master's degree. She was a serious student, studied hard, and was doing well. Sandra enrolled in a chemistry course requiring memorization of many symbols and formulas, as well as, analysis of complex scientific data. Though challenging, Sandra scored an 'A' on her first exam.

Ruth, also a 50ish woman, was enrolled in the same class. Soon after the exam, Ruth changed her classroom seat to sit next to Sandra. The two became friendly and often spent time together after class.

When Ruth asked for assistance with homework and writing assignments, Sandra always gave it. She was elated to have a school friend her age. It never occurred to Sandra that Ruth was using her.

The end of the semester arrived, along with the inevitable final exam. As the test was underway, Sandra caught Ruth copying from her. At one point, Ruth motioned instructions for Sandra to place her answer-sheet in a spot more conducive to Ruth's roaming eyes.

Sandra responded by repositioning her chair and her exam so Ruth could *not* see. Good move! Sandra had worked too hard to risk the chance of losing her college status for a cheat. (Cheating may lead to expulsion.) Sandra was enraged at Ruth for involving her in a situation that might jeopardize her education.

Would Ruth have struck up a friendship with Sandra if she did not get that first 'A?' We can only guess the true answer. Ruth stridently stated as long as Sandra had done the work and studied, she should share her knowledge (cheat) so Ruth could get a good grade.

Ruth's exact words were, 'I am too busy to study and it's no skin off your back if I also get an A.' Putting Sandra's pursuit of a Master's degree at risk did not enter Ruth's thinking. With Opera Singers nothing and no one ever does.

FRIENDSHIP STATUS
Ruth's response was hurtful, yet it was an eye-opener. Sandra realized she and Ruth were never really friends.

MOOCHING MINNIE
Looks for ways she can keep her money, while you spend yours – on her.

ROBIN'S STORY

Robin adored her friend Michelle. They had a lot in common and enjoyed each other's company. Their financial situations were similar. Neither had much disposable income, but as long as they kept tight budgets, they were all right.

Michelle kept to her budget by mooching off Robin. For

example, when they went out to eat, Michelle would claim lack of hunger and only order (and pay for) a drink and small salad. Then, she would eat a sizeable portion of Robin's meal (for which Robin was paying).

At times, Michelle would 'forget' her wallet and ask Robin to 'loan' her money for movies or another activity. Afterward, Robin felt awkward asking Michelle for repayment.

The situation became unbearable when Michelle steadily increased her uninvited visits to Robin's home – at dinnertime. Naturally, dropping by once in a while is acceptable, but Robin knew Michelle was intensifying her mooching. Robin had to address Michelle's actions before her resentment eroded the friendship.

Interestingly, Michelle's response to Robin was the same as Ruth's response to Sandra in the previous story. As long as Robin was cooking, Michelle reasoned, 'what is the big deal if I drop by at dinnertime?' Robin replied the big deal is she feels pressured to purchase and prepare extra food for Michelle. Robin no longer wanted that burden and expense.

The resolution: Robin proposed a weekly dinner. Each week they rotate hosting, planning, purchasing, and preparing a meal. Unless invited, there are no more spontaneous dinnertime visits.

After resolving this issue, Robin was reluctant to bring up the topic of restaurant meals. She put together a workable plan that did not require a major confrontation.

In the past, when the two friends ate out, Michelle used the 'I am not hungry' gimmick to limit her order (and payment). Miraculously, Michelle's hunger always materialized as soon as Robin's food was served – just in time to help herself to a hefty portion.

Following the new plan, as Robin and Michelle peruse restaurant menus, Robin asserts she is very hungry, intends to eat her entire meal, and does not want to share. Much to Robin's relief, after a few awkward attempts, Michelle finally got the message and began to order, and pay for, her own food.

Presently, Michelle is getting another message. Robin rebuffs Michelle's requests to be her personal ATM. If Michelle 'forgets' her wallet or 'does not have time' to get cash from the bank before the movie (or other activity) begins, Robin says, 'let's do something else.'

FRIENDSHIP STATUS
Mooching Michelle is no longer able to exploit Robin's generosity. Michelle is cranky. Too bad.

FOOD FOR THOUGHT

Be steadfast and consistent. The Triplets thrive on guilt and inconsistency.

2 THE SOB SISTERS FAMILY

Members of this family use their sad tales to excuse inexcusable behavior. We want to shout, 'No more excuses. Enough is enough.'

VIOLA THE VICTIM

The alpha member of The Sob Sisters Family is Viola The Victim. Time after time, Viola tells the same story of how life, family, relationships, work, yada, yada, yada, cause her to suffer.

The daily or weekly details may vary, meaning this week Viola's husband (brother, employer, colleague, stranger,) did this instead of that, but the gist of her sob story is the same old, same old. Viola is a one-tune song stuck on the poor me, pity me refrain.

At first, Viola's friends listen, commiserate, comfort, and advise. After weeks, months, and perhaps years, we finally *get* it. Viola refuses any and all guidance. She just wants others to listen to her tales of woe.

We are disturbed to think Viola opts to be a victim. How is it possible for Viola to *choose* this kind of life? Clearly, the reasons are complex and complicated. Rather than seeking solutions to her issues, Viola seeks attention and pity for her suffering. Can you feel your energy being drained?

FOOD FOR THOUGHT

Swamp Goddesses receive attention for being fabulous, not for being victims. When we have a problem, we search for the best possible outcome.

MORE FOOD FOR THOUGHT

Swamp Goddesses are loyal, wonderful friends. We are supportive and compassionate. Regrettably, a friendship with Viola The Victim is an unhealthy trap. Swamp Goddesses do not get sucked into traps that allow Viola to drain our energy.

REMINDER

Those of us going through menopausal mayhem and aging angst need our energy. Now is not the time to squander our supplies on emotional vampires.

NEEDY NELLY

Viola's sister is Needy Nelly. Have you met her? She is the one constantly calling us, whining, 'Where are you? I need you. I am falling. Pick me up. Now!' Different Nellys use different pleas, but the narrative is the same.

For Nelly, everything is a crisis. She dials our number because we are her 911. She calls at all hours. Nelly apparently does not care if we are working, sleeping, or rescuing our favorite shoe from the dog. Nelly demands we drop everything for her, no matter what we are doing.

FOOD FOR THOUGHT

Swamp Goddesses are there to pick up our friends when they fall. We are available in a crisis. However, Needy Nelly is always falling and she labels most things crises.

MORE FOOD FOR THOUGHT

Swamp Goddesses establish personal boundaries and respect the boundaries of others – friends included.

YVONNE'S STORY

Yvonne had a full, busy life. Nonetheless, she tried to be available for her childhood friend Myra. From the time they were very young, Myra counted on Yvonne to take care of her.

Yvonne grew accustomed to Myra's many phone calls filled with ongoing neediness. Then, Yvonne's double milestone patience level decreased and the strings tying the two friends together tugged tighter and tighter – until she felt strangled by them.

Yvonne attempted to set boundaries and limit Myra's 'emergency' calls. It was not easy to alter established patterns. Finally, Yvonne's weariness reached the breaking point. Yolanda told Myra she was no longer available 24/7. In fact, her new policy was to shut off the phone at 10PM.

Thinking she was clever, Myra found a way to circumvent Yvonne's new rule. She continued to call after 10PM. Instead of speaking with Yvonne, Myra spoke to Yvonne's voice mail. Myra said the sound of her friend's voice recording, coupled with the knowledge Yvonne will eventually hear Myra's problems, soothed her.

Oh goody. Just what we all want accompanying our morning cup of tea – a rambling report of Needy Nelly's nightly dramas.

The situation deteriorated after Yvonne began a serious relationship with a man. (She had been divorced for years.) If Yvonne did not answer the phone before the 10PM deadline, Myra not only stated her present Needy Nelly crisis, but also would try to figure out where Yvonne was and what she was doing. Myra declared (on voice mail) her assumptions of Yvonne's schedule and supposed whereabouts for the day. Creepy.

Yvonne had another talk with Myra. Yvonne explained why she could not handle Myra's Needy Nelly antics. To remain friends, Yvonne said they must have deference for each other's boundaries.

FRIENDSHIP STATUS
Yvonne and Myra are still working things through.

DUMPSTER DOTTIE
Dottie is Nelly's granddaughter. Dottie believes her friends are her private dumpster. Why should she carry around her problems when she can dump them on us? Dottie releases her burdens, feels relieved, and goes on her way – never thinking of those left to carry her load.

FOOD FOR THOUGHT

We have enough double milestone extra weight. We do not need Dottie's load added to our already increasing poundage. Ummmm ... bad joke?

DENISE'S STORY

Denise and Bonnie were close friends. The two women met the first day they began working for a large insurance company. They had lunch together every weekday, but did not see or speak to each other on weekends. Bonnie's abusive husband would not allow it.

Each week it was the same. Mondays, Denise listened as Bonnie recounted the horrors of time alone with her spouse. Fridays, Bonnie declared her dread of the upcoming weekend.

Denise wanted to *save* Bonnie. She offered advice on ways to end violent relationships. Denise located support services for abused women and presented her findings to Bonnie. In return, Bonnie gave vague excuses for staying with her husband. Sometimes, she defended him. Unfortunately, this is usual.

FRIENSHIP STATUS

Denise was trapped in a Dumpster Dottie friendship. As long as Bonnie was able to dump her troubles on Denise, she 'felt better.' Meanwhile, Denise felt worse. Denise spent her weekends burdened with worry and concern for Bonnie's well-being.

HELPFUL HINTS

Denise must initiate change. In a straightforward manner, Denise has to let Bonnie know she is ready and willing to provide support *after* Bonnie ends her relationship. Until then, Denise has no choice. Starting immediately, she becomes unavailable to hear tales of brutality. This course of action requires extraordinary fortitude, but it is necessary in order for Bonnie to save herself.

FOOD FOR THOUGHT

Bonnie's tales of abuse shock her friends. We cannot understand why Bonnie stays in a violent relationship. As with other Sob Sisters, the reasons why they are who they are, and do what they do, are complex and complicated.

MORE FOOD FOR THOUGHT

Swamp Goddesses never allow ourselves to be abused. No how, no way, not ever. If you're in a violent relationship, you deserve better. Professional support is available. Take care of yourself. Now.

For Swamp Goddesses in the process of releasing addictions, such as drinking alcohol, taking drugs, gambling, or other substances and behaviors – stay strong. Although recovery is an ongoing process, it's worth it. Everyone is rooting for you.

Many Swamp Goddesses have friends who are in recovery. We want to do what we can to bolster their healing. Each of us has to realistically decide how much energy we are willing to give. Be honest. Do not make promises you cannot keep. Set limits and stick to them.

NOT RECOVERING RENEE

Renee is a well-known member of The Sob Sisters Family. She differs from those who courageously and successfully face the challenges of recovery. Renee is on a path to *non-recovery.* It twists, turns, and leads back to nowhere.

Sob Sister Renee is full of unmet intentions and unfulfilled promises. Renee's addiction directly affects her friends when she pleads for things we are not comfortable giving, while always promising she will *never* again ask for anything. *Never* for Renee may be thirty minutes.

FOOD FOR THOUGHT

Addiction is allowing something or someone to control our lives. Swamp Goddesses control our lives. We do not give damaging, unhealthy substances and behaviors that power. If you have traveled the tortured path of addiction, enroll in a treatment program to guide your recovery. You can do it.

MORE FOOD FOR THOUGHT

Swamp Goddesses' cravings are centered on life-affirming, healthy behaviors, such as having as much joy, love, and light in our lives as possible … and chocolate.

3 THE GREENS

At first sight, we assume The Green Family is comprised of environmentalists turning green to express their ideology. Not! The green color of this Family reflects their main personality trait – envy. It underlies most of what they do.

GRETA THE GREEN GOBLIN

Greta is the head mistress of The Green Family. She is always watching and weighing what her friends have and what she does not. Deprivation underscores Greta's mindset.

Greta can't genuinely celebrate her friends' joyous occasions. She reacts to her friends' good news by feeling deprived and jealous. Greta is not sincere in praising our accomplishments. In response to whatever we achieve – from the well-deserved promotion at work, the birth of our delicious grandbabies, or finally losing 20 lbs – Greta turns a gruesome green.

Expert-level Gretas are specialists at bizarrely twisting their friends' triumphs. The result is we console Greta and downplay our happiness because it arrives while she *suffers.* This Greta achieves top scores on Masterful Maneuvers.

FOOD FOR THOUGHT

Don't give Greta the power to diminish your happiness.

Other members of The Green Family are NEGATIVE NAN, CRITICAL CATHY and DOOMSDAY DORA. We know this group. The threesome display ardent jealousy by finding fault with what we say and do.

For this trio, anything and everything comes under their harsh scrutiny. With a comment or glance, they disapprove of all – including our occupation, spouse, shoes, and recent choice of vacation destination. Isn't it time to tell them to 'stuff it?'

FOOD FOR THOUGHT

There is a substantial difference between constructive criticism evidenced by caring, doable tips and destructive criticism purposely meant to tear us down and cause pain.

MORE FOOD FOR THOUGHT

Swamp Goddesses rejoice for, and with, our friends. Most importantly, we are prudent with our advice and only give it when asked. This requires practice.

HELEN'S STORY

Helen is a recently retired teacher. Throughout Helen's teaching career, she spent her rare free time crafting beautiful jewelry. Retirement gave Helen the opportunity to open a jewelry design business. After 35 years dedicated to educating young children, she is excited to get on with life's next chapter. Things are going well.

Things are not going well for Helen's former colleague, Rita. She has years left before being eligible for her own retirement.

The two women became friends while working at the same school. They shared the highs and lows that accompany a teaching career. Rita misses their daily ritual of summing up the day's victories and disappointments.

Helen wants to continue the friendship with Rita. Helen likes to sporadically reminisce, but she has no interest in everyday teaching related discussions. Helen is concentrating on her future, not her past.

Rita is concentrating on jealousy of her friend's joy. Helen refuses to stand for it. Rita's disparaging remarks concerning Helen's studio, jewelry designs, and hard-won clients are unacceptable.

As a former teacher, Helen is an expert in addressing childish behavior. She puts on her best *teacher face*, uses her sturdy *teacher voice*, and scolds Rita for her offensive attitude. In order for their friendship to survive, Rita must 'grow up.'

Rita's jealousy is unmasked. She admits her true feelings concerning Helen's transformed life. Rita feels unhappily 'stuck' and wants what Helen has. Rita confesses she resorts to criticism and negativity when she's envious.

FRIENDSHIP STATUS

Rita knows Helen is a no-nonsense person. If Rita values the friendship, she will have to change her attitude. It remains to be seen whether or not Rita will (can) do that.

4 THE ANNOYING FAMILY

The Annoying Family is extensive. Each and every one of them snaps our last nerve.

ANGRY ANNIE

On most surveys, Annie is voted the most annoying member of her Family. Annie is furious at the world. She uses her anger as a weapon to manipulate everyone around her. No one wants to incur her wrath. This gives Annie power she has not earned and certainly doesn't deserve.

FOOD FOR THOUGHT

Angry Annie is a bully. If she gets angry, huff and puff and blow her house down. It is made of straw. Swamp Goddesses do not bully others, nor do we let others bully us.

PEGGY'S STORY

Linda was an abused child, then an abused wife. Even at her workplace, Linda disclosed personal stories to nearly all the people she met. According to friends and colleagues, Linda used this disclosure as a scheme to excuse her volatile tirades.

Peggy was Linda's office mate. They had to get along to go along. Peggy conceded precious office space, deferred to Linda's quirky requests, and walked on the proverbial eggshells. Peggy felt her unspoken job description included going out of her way to deflect any situation that would cause an outburst from Linda.

Peggy's accommodation approach did a turn-around the day her young grandchild came to visit. Peggy's grandson broke one of Linda's knickknacks. They both apologized to Linda and were extremely conciliatory.

True to form, Linda went ballistic. Then, she made a huge mistake. She dared to turn her fury on Peggy's grandson. It was as if time stopped. Peggy went into protective Grandma mode, got in Linda's face, and told her to, 'back off and '***' (Use your imagination to fill in the *colorful* words Peggy yelled in her granny rant.) Don't you love feisty women?

FRIENDSHIP STATUS
Peggy's perspective shifted after this incident. She was done catering to Linda's bullying exploitation. Impressive.

FOOD FOR THOUGHT

Don't mess with grandmothers. Aging does not stop women from being intense protectors, especially concerning children and grandchildren.

MORE FOOD FOR THOUGHT

As a rule, it is improper to publicize very personal subjects in the workplace.

ALWAYS RIGHT ROBERTA and her mother KNOW IT ALL NOREEN are prominent members of The Annoying Family. Roberta and Noreen think they have expertise in all areas. According to these two, they know everything; just ask them. The mother and daughter *geniuses* (again, just ask them), claim their knowledge ranges from interpreting Plato and deciphering arcane tax codes to adroitly wrapping gifts and efficiently preparing gourmet meals.

Noreen has the inside information concerning recent movies we watched or restaurants where we ate. She takes over our anecdotes. Annoying, but harmless.

Roberta is nasty. If anyone disagrees with her so-called knowledge, opinions, and thoughts, Roberta responds by telling us we are either uninformed, ignorant, or a terrible friend.

Roberta perceives disagreements as personal attacks. With this friendship, we must fight to have our knowledge, opinions, and thoughts respected.

FOOD FOR THOUGHT

Swamp Goddesses are secure in our intelligence. We do not compete with friends on brainpower contests. Nor do we hide our intelligence. That is ludicrous.

LAURA'S STORY

Florence is an Always Right Roberta. Whenever her friend Laura raised a topic, Florence knew all about it. This trait annoyed Laura, but she overlooked it because of the other qualities Florence brought to the friendship.

Laura's husband got ill. As the illness progressed, Laura and her husband consulted various medical specialists to determine the best treatment options.

Without being asked, Florence suggested a treatment different from what the doctors prescribed. Laura thanked Florence, but stated she and her husband were following the experts' recommendations.

Appallingly, Florence again pushed her idea and then complained that Laura's repeated rejection hurt her feelings. Obviously, Laura was in no mood to smooth over Florence's petulance. She told Florence to stop pressuring her. Laura needed to focus on her husband and did not have the time or emotional resources to pay attention to Florence's feelings.

No, Florence is not a medical authority. This is an incomprehensible case of a Know It All Noreen confident she knows more than the health care professionals.

FRIENDSHIP STATUS
When the crisis with Laura's husband passed, Florence was the one to end the friendship. She was 'insulted' by Laura's refusal to utilize her treatment proposal. What planet is she living on?

I HAVE BEEN THERAPIZED THEODORA
Some of us decide to try therapy as a way to resolve personal issues. Usually, this brings good results. Therapized Theodora exemplifies individuals (relatively few), who go into therapy and then behave in ways that challenge their friends' patience. Obviously, this is not a good result.

One bothersome characteristic of Therapized Theodora is her belief that, because she has been to therapy, she has gained the ability to analyze her friends. Theodora brazenly probes our psyches and dispenses unsolicited gibberish

FOOD FOR THOUGHT

We may not want to be confronted with our issues, or her perception of our issues. It is none of Theodora's business.

EMMA THE EMPRESS OF ENTITLEMENT
Therapized Theodora morphs into Emma when she unleashes - on everyone - her overblown sense of entitlement. Emma insists it compensates for all the pre-therapy years she did not feel entitled.

FOOD FOR THOUGHT

True healing means we do not take out our pain on friends, or expect them to service our newly obtained sense of entitlement. We are all Goddesses. Swamp Goddesses treat each other royally.

CARLY'S STORY

Carly's friend Teresa lived her life as a victim. Teresa was renowned for terribly bad choices that led to incredibly worse consequences.

Teresa entered therapy as a way to transform her decision-making skills. She rapidly began a personality makeover. Most of the changes were terrific; several were not. According to Carly, Teresa still had a few distorted sensibilities. When she was stressed, Teresa replaced poor choices with excessive demands.

For a while, Carly tried to put up with her friend's annoying behavior. When Carly's tolerance level stretched beyond repair, she told Teresa to, 'get over herself.'

FRIENDSHIP STATUS
This did not turn out well for the relationship. On the plus side, the ruined friendship motivated Teresa to continue therapy until she achieved more balance.

FOOD FOR THOUGHT

Therapy has a role in healing emotional wounds and traumas. A skilled therapist can guide us to relinquish unhealthy, possibly destructive behavioral patterns and adopt healthy, constructive ones.

NOTE

A few therapists get upset at stories of therapy patients gone awry. No reason to be upset.

LYING LOLA

Lola lies, lies, and then lies some more. Why does she lie? We may never know why, but we do know Lola's dishonesty is exasperating.

Sometimes, our Lola friends fabricate elaborate tales and expect us to cover for them. Back in high school, many of us covered for friends when they were spending time with forbidden boyfriends, skipping school, or doing other prohibited activities. That was then, and it seemed so exciting. This is now, and it is so annoying.

Do you want a liar for a friend? Have you convinced yourself Lola's other qualities make up for her dishonesty? What is your plan when Lola deceives you? Do not be fooled into believing you are exempt. When Lola lies about other people to us, it's guaranteed that Lola is lying about us to others. A liar is a liar.

FOOD FOR THOUGHT

Swamp Goddesses do not lie, nor are we complicit in any one else's lies. Swamp Goddesses realize deception comes naturally to Lola. She stretches the truth with ease.

FRAN'S STORY

Fran was friends with Stacy. They shared a lot in common, except for Stacy's relentless dishonesty. Fran believed, because they were best friends, Stacy did not lie to her or about her.

Yeah, right.

Fran frequently helped Stacy hide purchases of expensive clothes. Stacy used Fran's house to rip price tags off new items and discard shopping bags. Afterward, Stacy went home to her husband, seemingly empty-handed. If Stacy's husband detected a recent purchase, she fibbed and claimed it was borrowed from Fran.

Fran convinced herself omission is not a lie. Fran also convinced herself that Stacy's complaints about her husband were true. According to Stacy, her husband was stingy, controlled their money with an iron fist, and prevented Stacy from buying anything without his permission.

FRIENDSHIP STATUS

As it turned out, Fran learned nothing Stacy said about her husband was accurate. Stacy was hiding purchases with a number of people. Stacy's compulsive shopping and unrestrained spending pushed her family's already rocky financial situation straight into bankruptcy. Why does anyone trust a known liar?

AVOIDANCE AVA

Ava is Lola's niece. They both lie, but in different ways. Ava uses deception to avoid saying, 'I do not like this,' 'I can not do that,' or simply, 'no.'

Ava is well-intentioned, but misguided when she tells us what she thinks we want to hear – our haircut looks stylish (it is much too short), our swimsuit fits well (actually it reveals an abundance of jiggly stuff), or she is free to attend a concert with us next weekend. (Ava is already booked for something else.)

Ava's unreliability is easy to observe. How can it not be? Ava repeatedly makes soon-to-be unfulfilled promises. Does she think we will not notice when her promises don't come through? Ava has no credibility.

FOOD FOR THOUGHT

If we ask for an opinion, we don't want lies. Or, do we? Do we really want to know the truth all the time, about everything?

MORE FOOD FOR THOUGHT

Swamp Goddesses are honest with ourselves and with others. On second thought … maybe it is not necessary to know how much jiggly stuff is hanging out of our swimwear.

ANDREA"S STORY

Andrea wanted to be liked. She invested a lot of effort into creating an image of being a kind and thoughtful person. This is a noble ambition. Andrea mistakenly believed she could reinforce this lofty image by saying 'yes' to all requests for favors. Anyone who has made it to adulthood knows this strategy is destined for failure.

Before Andrea's menopausal mayhem and aging angst reared their ugly double heads, friends and family always depended on her. After the double milestone, Andrea's *Never Say No* image began to crumble. She found it difficult to follow through with her numerous commitments. Yet, Andrea refused to even murmur the magic 'no' word.

It took time for Andrea to realize she not only spoiled her family and friends, but also unintentionally trained them to take advantage of her. Andrea's watershed moment arrived the day she committed to three appointments, each for the same time. Why would she do this? Because 'no' was not in Andrea's vocabulary.

Andrea convinced herself she could do all three. She did try. Just as Andrea dropped off a friend at a doctor's appointment, she had to drive her son to the airport. By that time, Andrea missed the major event – a job interview.

It took a bit of introspection and reflection for Andrea to understand why she worked so hard to never say 'no' and also, come to terms with the futility of 'buying' affection.

Eventually, she began to modify her ways. Soon after becoming a budding Swamp Goddess, Andrea accepted the word 'no' into her vocabulary. From then on, Andrea committed only to things she was *able* to do.

When she became a full-fledged Swamp Goddess, Andrea committed only to things she *wanted* to do. This left a number of people disappointed. They could no longer take advantage of her. Boo Hoo.

STATUS UPDATE
Now, her real friends appreciate that when Andrea says 'yes,' she means it. This works well for Andrea and everyone currently in her life.

BLABBERMOUTH BETTY
Betty is a non-stop blabber. Nothing we say to Betty is sacred. She promises secrecy, does pinkie swears, and takes vows of silence on the lives of her loved ones. None of it matters. Betty cannot control herself. She tells all. Never fall for Betty's assurances to keep secrets. She will not.

FOOD FOR THOUGHT

Swamp Goddesses hold confidences. Swamp Goddesses know it is naïve to believe Betty will keep our secrets while she is sharing another friend's secrets with us. We are ready to wake up and smell the gossip.

EVEYLN'S STORY

Evelyn bubbled with excitement when her daughter phoned with wonderful news. She was pregnant with twins. Evelyn's daughter wanted to keep her pregnancy private until the first trimester passed. Most expectant couples do this.

Justine overheard the call from Evelyn's daughter. Evelyn worried because Justine is an unrepentant gossiper. Justine's friends have learned never, ever to tell her anything significant. She is careless with their personal information.

Evelyn pleaded with Justine to honor her daughter's request for privacy. Justine agreed and then, almost immediately, demonstrated why she earned her nickname, Blabbermouth Betty. Within a few hours, Justine blabbed the pregnancy details to several people who, in turn, contacted Evelyn to congratulate her.

FRIENDSHIP STATUS

When confronted by Evelyn, Justine defended her broken promise by stating, 'I told everyone it is a secret and not to tell.' Classic Blabbermouth.

LATE AGAIN LAVERNE

Laverne is habitually late and her friends have run out of patience. How annoying is Laverne? How maddening is waiting for Laverne? How much time has been wasted waiting for Laverne? The real question is, why are we asking *how* while still waiting for Laverne?

Laverne cites lack of time-management skills. Laverne expects friends to have empathy for her inability to correctly calculate how long it takes to get ready or to estimate the correct distance to her destination.

When Laverne is late, she makes excuses, apologizes, and assures her friends it will not happen again. We know otherwise. Let's be candid. Laverne has blatant disregard for our time.

Many friends have attempted to *fix* Laverne's tardiness. A common ploy is to *fudge the facts.* For example, we say the movie begins at 7PM, but it actually begins at 8PM. The problem with this scheme is obvious. It can be used only until Laverne figures out our ruse and is back to usual.

It is rude and disrespectful to cause others to wait. Do you have Laverne friends who dismiss your complaints with, 'Pul-eeze, it is only twenty minutes?' Yes, but that is twenty minutes of our lives, multiplied by the zillions of minutes we have previously been kept waiting, and will continue to be kept waiting. No thanks.

WANDA'S STORY

Wanda and Jane met as moms with small children. Although their children had grown and moved away, Wanda and Jane remained friends. Wanda prided herself on being prompt. No matter if business or personal, Wanda was punctual for all appointments. In contrast, Jane was always late.

When the kids were small, Jane's lateness was irritating, but given their hectic lives, Wanda let it pass. As one consequence of Wanda's menopausal misery and aging angst, she decided to respect her precious time and stop waiting for Jane.

If they scheduled a get-together and Jane did not arrive on time, Wanda went forward with their planned activity. When the two of them were supposed to see a movie, Wanda went into the theatre by herself. As usual, Jane missed the beginning scenes, but it no longer affected Wanda's enjoyment of the entire movie.

After a while, Wanda came up with an improved strategy. Now, she only makes plans with Jane if others are involved. When Jane is late for dinners, concerts, or hikes, Wanda takes off with her other companions. Based on Jane's history, the friends give a measly five-minute grace period. If she is not there, they leave. It's Jane's loss.

FRIENDSHIP STATUS

In a sappy movie, this story would end with Jane learning her lesson and arriving on time for all future outings. Instead, we get the real story. Jane continues being late and missing opportunities to have fun with friends. Again, her loss.

FOOD FOR THOUGHT

Swamp Goddesses value our time and the time of others. We respect friends and colleagues by being prompt. Life intervenes for everyone, of course, and there are instances when we are late. We get delayed by unexpected traffic, sidelined with an urgent call, or mired in a last minute work issue. With this in mind, Swamp Goddesses make time allowances for the unexpected.

MORE FOOD FOR THOUGHT

If you choose to use Wanda's policy – good for you. You are valuing yourself by valuing your time.

REMINDER

The policy works best if used consistently.

NOSY NADINE

Personal boundaries do not exist for Nadine. She is in our business all the time. She pokes into our closets, drawers, and medicine cabinets. She has been caught reading our mail.

Some Nosy Nadines ask very personal questions that shake our comfort zone. She wants intimate details of our marriage struggles, salary negotiations, and sibling rivalries. When she asks us to disclose our weight, then we know she is totally out of control.

FOOD FOR THOUGHT

Swamp Goddesses are upfront about comfort zones. We state our limits, but we're not obliged to justify them.

STEPHANIE'S STORY

Stephanie is a recuperating nosy person. She believed her friends had the inside scoop on everything. This explained why they supposedly knew more than she did, from exclusive shopping sites to mysterious sexual techniques. Her distorted notions led to Stephanie's inappropriate questions and meddlesome activities.

Stephanie's two closest friends arranged an informal *intervention*. They told Stephanie she was busted. The two women liked Stephanie, but had enough of her prying. Stephanie was given an ultimatum. If Stephanie did not stop snooping, they would stop – being friends with her.

This had an immediate impact on Stephanie. She listened to what her friends said. Early into the *intervention*, Stephanie acknowleded her nosiness was a feeble attempt to ascertain her friends' 'secrets' in order to figure out how to be just like them.

FRIENDSHIP STATUS
Stephanie decided to examine her deep feelings of insecu-

rity. Her friends encouraged these efforts and were constant sources of support. This is a good story.

SARA THE SCOREKEEPER

Sara The Scorekeeper keeps a running tally. If we ask for
a favor, almost instantaneously, she requests a favor in
return. Sara tests our friendship by demanding a *huge*
favor. As a result, we are unwilling to ask anything of Sa-
rah. The payback is too costly.

FOOD FOR THOUGHT

*Friends do each other favors. This is a given. With friend-
ships based on reciprocity, the favors tend to even out –
especially when measured over the length of the relationship. Swamp Goddesses trust in that. Sara The Scorekeeper
does not.*

KELLY'S STORY

Kelly sold her house and moved to an apartment in a different part of town. She was delighted to meet Allison. They became friendly. This helped Kelly's transition, not only to her
new community, but also to her new life as a widow.

Kelly went away for a few days to visit her daughter. Before
leaving, Kelly asked Allison to feed her bird – sprinkle some
food into the birdcage. Allison agreed.

When Kelly arrived home from her trip, Allison had an idea

for 'payback.' She wanted Kelly to keep her dog – for a week! Allison claimed she needed a break from the constant walking and caretaking that dogs require. Did I mention it was wintertime?

Kelly was in a bind. She suspected Allison was testing her. Kelly wanted to continue the friendship with Allison, but a week of dogsitting was too much of a burden for her.

Kelly reversed Allison's friendship test by telling the truth and letting Allison know there were limits to the favors she was willing to do. Allison said she understood Kelly's position and was 'okay' with it. This remains to be seen. Kelly will never again ask Allison for a favor.

FRIENDSHIP STATUS
Shaky.

FOOD FOR THOUGHT

Owing debts to Scorekeepers is costly.

5 THE SCARED, SCARY, SUDDENLY SINGLE FAMILY

This family is comprised of recently divorced and widowed folks who are terrified of being without a mate. They have an intense fear of being alone and living alone.

The anticipation of living life solo is terrifying for the freshly divorced or widowed. It is quite understandable, and actually expected, to feel unsure and frightened. After being part of a couple, these folks have to adapt to a different lifestyle.

Although new singles may dislike their unfamiliar status, most are resilient enough to make the necessary adjustment. After a while, quite a few widows and divorcees are pleasantly surprised at how much they enjoy their own space. Many genuinely thrive, especially if they distinguish the difference between being alone and being lonely.

In fact, some singles get so comfortable with their new independence, they will not give it up – even if presented with alternative arrangements. Living alone provides the unique opportunity to do what we want, when we want – a defining Swamp Goddess attitude.

More importantly, once double milestoners master the ability to be alone, we're free to selectively choose our partners – if we want one – not, need one. Swamp Goddesses have high standards. It is always a mistake to lower them.

FOOD FOR THOUGHT

If you're sure you do not want to live by yourself, ask a friend or family member to share your home. This is infinitely better than desperately seeking almost anyone to fill the 'emptiness.'

ALONEAPHOBE ALANA, DESPERATE DELORES and GAIL THE GOODBYE GIRL

These are three scary, scared, suddenly single cousins. It is scary to observe how the scared cousins set about to change their new status. None of the three takes time to heal from her loss. This leads to serious consequences as the cousins become scarier and scarier.

As we watch with horror, Aloneaphobe Alana applies no standards for potential partners. Desperate Dolores becomes frightening and frightful as we witness her doing anything to be part of a couple. Gail The Goodbye Girl is so frantic for a replacement relationship, she believes all her attention must be directed toward finding, and then keeping, a man – lest he slips away.

When Gail enters into a relationship, she says goodbye to her friends. There is no room for friends in Gail's highly prized, coupled-up life. This behavior was not cool in adolescence and is totally repugnant in midlife.

MARIA'S STORY

Maria has three grown daughters. As soon as the youngest daughter left home, she and her husband of 35 years divorced. Divorce meant Maria had to live alone. She never had this experience. Maria shared a home with her parents and siblings until her wedding day. She then lived with her husband and, eventually, children.

Maria did not give herself time to adjust to single life. Three weeks! after the separation, Maria began a frantic search for a man to fill her perceived 'empty space.' She had no aspiration of filling up herself. Maria wanted a man to do it. As it turned out, any man.

Maria reconnected with someone from the past. This person was blatant evidence of her desperation. Maria's new (old) friend was insecure and needy. These characteristics were manifested as jealousy and possessiveness. Added to the warning signals, Maria's *boyfriend* was threatened by her friends, especially her single friends.

Throughout her difficult marriage and divorce, Maria relied on a closely-knit network of both married and single women for comfort and companionship. Maria was so determined to provide solid evidence of loyalty to *loser* man, she actually dropped these friends in a foolish attempt to prove … what? Her friends wonder to what extent Maria will grovel? Next, will Maria give up her children, her brother?

FRIENDSHIP STATUS

Maria assumes her friends will be there if (when) this relationship ends. Probably not. At first, Maria's friends were bewildered; soon thereafter they became angry. In due course, the friends felt various levels of repulsion at the enduring images of Maria's desperation.

FOOD FOR THOUGHT

Desperation is neither a worthy motivation nor a sound foundation for a strong, loving relationship. Swamp Goddesses are romantic, yet rational. No matter how blissful a blossoming romance may be, it is a Blaring Red Alert when we are asked to sacrifice our family and friends. Run!

MORE FOOD FOR THOUGHT

Both romance and friendship enrich our lives. Swamp Goddesses find ways for friends and romantic partners to coexist.

CHAPTER 7

THE SWAMP GODDESS FRIENDSHIP ASSESSMENT (SGFA)

PART C – INITIAL REACTIONS

OBJECTIVE
To survey SGFA Portion 1 Initial Reactions

DIRECTIONS
Use paper and pen to record your responses.

✪ Describe your reactions to the personalities described in Chapter 6.

✪ Do you recognize any of The Families? Which ones seem most familiar?

FOOD FOR THOUGHT

If you do not have any friends with the loathsome person-alities described in Chapter 6, your friends likely come from Families, such as: Wise Wonderful Women, Gracious Glorious Gals, Fun Fab Femmes, Kind Caring Crew, Legendary Lovely Ladies, and Honorable Dames of Integrity.

Congratulations. You choose your friends well. Give yourself a big Swamp Goddess hug.

For those who have friends from notorious Families, join the club. That's just about all of us. We are ready to make changes in order to improve our current friendships and create quality new ones. Yippee!

MY STORY

In my pre-Swamp Goddess life, I carelessly squandered energy. Like many of you, taking care of others took priority over taking care of myself.

Consequently, I *attracted* self absorbed, energy draining Opera Singers who endlessly repeated the 'I, I, I, Me, Me, Me' refrain. Conversely, they were *attracted* to me because they wanted one-sided relationships. We were well-matched characters playing out dysfunctional nightmares … until I had an unexpected quarrel with an Opera Singer friend.

Interestingly, the argument occurred a few days after the birth of Swamp Goddess. I do not wonder whether luck, fate, or random coincidence played a role in the two almost simultaneous events. It does not matter. What matters most – and what I am truly grateful for – is that both led me to scrutinize, and then transform, my relationships and, ultimately, my life.

The friendship-altering quarrel was accompanied by a jolting Swamp Goddess *ah-ha* moment. It was as if my friend's behavior prodded me to snap out of an Opera Singer-induced coma. As I recount the incident, it seems incredible this really happened. It did.

The saga began when a friend got angry because I refused her *demand* to 'come first' in my life. My newly bestowed Swamp Goddess self became electrified with a burst of indignation. It was ridiculous to be in the position of *ranking* people. But, my friend asked and I answered. Emphatically, I *placed* her after my actual priorities – family (and others). I knew the foundation of this friendship was permanently shattered, but I was left with nagging questions.

How did this person get such a distorted sense of our relationship? Why did a friend think she had primacy in my life, especially over my actual priorities?

Did I contribute to her deluded thinking? What signals was I sending to her, and other friends, that left room for misinterpretation?

It was unsettling that someone I considered a friend had such a warped vision of our friendship. Her assumption forced me to take an in-depth look at how and why I attracted an obvious Opera Singer into my life. Were there more? I cringe to admit there were plenty. After doing the necessary self-examination, I gladly let go of each and every Opera Singer.

The good news – they are not missed.

The great news – With energy draining Opera Singers banished, I began to feel the rewards of protecting, respecting, and utilizing my energy in healthy ways. It has been wonderful.

YOUR STORY

I know you have at least one special story.

Add it here.

_____

_____

_____

_____

_____

_____

_____

_____

_____

_____

_____

_____

_____

_____

_____

_____

FOOD FOR THOUGHT

Turn The Swamp Goddess Lens on yourself and answer this tough question.

• Do you fit any of The Family member descriptions from Chapter 6? Specify and elaborate.

HELPFUL HINT

Self-examination is intense, but the resulting awareness is well worth it.

CHAPTER 8

THE SWAMP GODDESS FRIENDSHIP ASSESSMENT (SGFA)

PART D – EVALUATION

OBJECTIVES
To identify personality patterns

To establish friendship criteria

To decide each friend's status

DESCRIPTION
After viewing personality types through The Swamp Goddess Lens, we begin assessing our friendships.

❀ This is you being proactive – excellent.

❀ This is you owning your life – very excellent.

DIRECTIONS

Use pen and paper to record your responses.

Review the personalities within each Family.

Review your list of friends.

Match friends and personalities.

Do any of your friends match the personality types described in Chapter 6?

☻ Are your friends spread evenly among The Families? Or, are your friends clustered in one or two Families?

☻ List each friend and her matching Family or Families.

☻ Why do you think you're friends with these personality types?

Do any of the following reasons hold true for you?

☻ A friend's personality reminds you of someone from childhood, e.g. parent, sibling, uncle, etc.

☻ The friendship fulfills a need. If so, what need, e.g. obligation, pity?

☻ What exactly is the obligation? What is the source of the pity?

☻ Unsure.

HELPFUL HINTS

Set your own pace. Get a dose of caffeine – coffee, tea, chocolate. Do a few stretches. Or, take as many power naps as needed.

MORE HELPFUL HINTS

If it is more manageable, narrow the list and focus on your three closest friends. Later, go back and finish the process for the remaining friends on your list.

FOOD FOR THOUGHT

The evaluation portion of The SGFA is designed to promote awareness. This is a central step in making wise choices and, ultimately, owning our lives. Attraction to either positive or negative personality types is highlighted.

In this context, *attraction* means we are drawn, or pulled, to certain character traits. In most cases, we are not consciously aware this is happening. If the pull is to positive, we have reason to celebrate.

If the pull is to negative, we have reason to feel concern. Negative *attraction* is perplexing, especially when we know interactions with these personalities are frequently hurtful.

Theories abound suggesting why certain people come into our lives, particularly why we seem to repeatedly *attract* individuals with similar positive or negative characteristics.

FOOD FOR THOUGHT

Theories are not facts. You can believe and agree with them or doubt and reject them. Your decision.

Here are a couple of *attraction* theories.

⊛ A particular personality type is recognizable and reminds us of individuals from our childhood.

When we were young and impressionable, we formed patterns of interacting with people (in our lives by circumstance, not choice) who had certain traits. In adulthood, we get involved with these same personality types, repeating familiar patterns – even if negative, even if painful. That is, until we do what needs to be done to release the *attraction*.

⊛ To provide opportunities for us to learn *lessons*

Doing an assessment of friendships, or any personal associations, is analogous to staring long and hard into a mirror. When we take a close look, the relationship we have with ourselves is reflected back in the faces of those we *attract* into our lives and their behavior toward us. Huh???

Simply stated, the way we treat ourselves is the way others treat us. We give cues, mostly inadvertently – some verbal, many not – which behaviors we accept and endure, as well as, those we do not. Thus, we teach people how to behave toward us.

For example, if we don't pay attention to ourselves and re-peatedly ignore our personal needs, we *attract* folks who do not pay attention to us and ignore our needs. If we dis-respect ourselves, we *attract* folks who disrespect us.

When we treat ourselves with attention and respect, we *attract* individuals who treat us with attention and respect (as well as other magnificent goodies). Anything less is un-acceptable and intolerable. In other words, the way we expect to be treated is broadcast loudly and clearly on all channels. Everyone receives the message. Sounds good.

There is one critical caveat to this theory. Faking, acting *as if,* or any other inauthentic behavior, doesn't work. If we don't authentically honor ourselves, or genuinely know we are worthy of being treated superbly, our message will not be sent or received clearly. Instead, it will be sent and re-ceived as static on the line.

FOOD FOR THOUGHT

This isn't at all about blaming the victim. Don't go there. It is about gaining insight into why we make certain choices, while simultaneously claiming the choices (and their pre-dictable results) are not what we want.

REMINDER

Insight is a step to wise decision-making and taking con-trol of our lives.

NOTE

This chapter skimmed the surface of complex issues. It is beyond the scope of *Help! I Surrounded By Bitches ...* to elaborate further. Nonetheless, if you are interested in delving more deeply into *attraction*, or other theories, sharpen your critical thinking skills and go for it.

Broadening your knowledge is a way to honor, respect, and love yourself. All are powerful components of The Swamp Goddess lifestyle.

Some of us pursue counseling as a way to clarify this complicated topic. Getting help is sending yourself the message you are worth it. Think of counseling as a priceless gift from you to you.

PROCEED TO THE SWAMP GODDESS FRIENDSHIP ASSESSMENT PORTION 2. (Appendix A)

CHAPTER 9

DECISIONS, DECISIONS, DECISIONS

DESCRIPTION

After completing The Swamp Goddess Friendship Assessment (Portions 1 & 2), The Keepers and The Dumpees will be evident. The Keepers are the friends you undoubtedly know to keep and The Dumpees are those you definitely know to let go.

There probably will be friends who fit into The Unsure category. They will require more attention. Thus, an entire chapter is devoted to Unsures (See Chapter 11).

First, let's start with the easy part. Uhhh… relatively easy.

DIRECTIONS

Use pen and paper to record your responses.

✪ List The Keepers. These are the friends you have decided to keep in your life.

✪ Next to each name write why you have selected them for this category

✪ List The Dumpees. These are the friends you have decided to let go.

✪ Next to each name write why you have selected them for this category.

FOOD FOR THOUGHT

If you have more than three names on the Keeper List – Wow. Most of us will be lucky to have one or two.

Do not get rattled if you have more names on The Dump List than on The Keeper List. That result is to be expected when we reach the double milestone. It is a by-product of our journey through the friendship frenzy of menopausal mayhem and aging angst.

CAUTION!

With the onset of the double milestone, many of us have become exquisitely sensitive to real or perceived slights. As difficult as it is to believe, from time to time, all of us can be unpleasant and obnoxious. (I know. It's shocking to confess such things.)

Be aware of your newly minted friendship scrutiny. Take care to distinguish between a one-time (or rare) unpleasant incident from an otherwise solid, precious friend and ongoing, annoying behavior that occurs regularly.

There is no need – after a single action – to tag a friend as an Angry Annie, Opportunistic Opal, Sara the Scorekeeper, or any other insufferable character. It is when actions are consistent and constant, that a friend, along with her routine behavior, classifies as one of the personalities outlined in Chapter 6.

CHLOE'S STORY

Chloe and Jane trace their friendship back to the day they were assigned as college roommates. Now, thirty years later, their bond remains strong and dependable. Life has been good for both women. They have solid marriages, happy adult children, and successful careers.

Last year, a wrinkle was thrown into Jane's life. Her father was diagnosed with Alzheimer's disease. Jane was crushed by her dad's illness and relied on Chloe's steadfast support. Chloe listened to each detail from the initial diagnosis, through the revolving doors of doctors, and finally to options for hospice facilities.

Recently, for no apparent reason, Chloe fell into a funk and was feeling blue. She mentioned her mood to Jane. Instead of the usual supportive shoulder to lean on, Jane chastised Chloe for 'complaining' and dismissed Chloe's feelings with 'go watch a movie.'

Jane's cavalier response infuriated Chloe, especially after almost a full year of seemingly one-sided conversations focused on Jane and her dad. Chloe was a hair's breath

away from descending into full friendship frenzy and im-
petuously severing her connection with Jane.

Good sense took hold and Chloe chose to talk out her feelings with Jane. Chloe told Jane she was hurt by her words
and her tone. Jane was horrified. She never meant to of-
fend Chloe. Was it Jane's menopausal mayhem and aging
angst acting up that day? Or, had the two women been
friends for so long, they took each other for granted?

FRIENDSHIP STATUS
Chloe and Jane had no intention of letting go of this special friendship. They pledged to tell each other whenever
they feel offended by something the other says or does.
Uh-huh. This can get verrrry interesting.

CHAPTER 10

ENDINGS

After completing SGFA Portions 1&2, we are face-to-face with the reality of ending friendships. Our newly acquired skills include: identifying personalities we attract, friendship qualities and common ground traits we rate important, plus those we label intolerable.

All this adds up to distinguishing between what we want and do not want – our personal Swamp Goddess Friendship Criteria. As a result, now we know the friends to keep and those to let go.

Ending a friendship is equivalent to breaking up with a romantic partner. We sputter overused phrases, such as, 'this is not working,' 'we have nothing in common,' 'you have changed,' 'I have changed,' and other musty, worn-out clichés.

For some endings, we choose silence and let the friendship die from neglect. We pretend to be unavailable to spend time together or to talk on the phone. In my younger years, I denounced this option as disrespectful and cowardly. I have since changed my mind, or shall I say, flip-flopped (good thing I am not a politician). Rarely are any of us eager for a big deal breakup, especially now.

FALLOUT

Regardless of the way in which our breakup with a friend occurs, it affects others. Usually, we were part of a large group or shared a couple of mutual friends. The breakup of our relationship creates tricky dilemmas for those other friends.

Some mutual friends may feel compelled to take sides. It is fine if friends take our side, but what if they do the unthinkable and, instead, take our (now) non-friend's side. Ouch!

In a worst-case scenario, mutual friends take the ex-friend's side, form alliances, shut us out, and we lose these friends as well. Double ouch!

FOOD FOR THOUGHT

When we ended a friendship, we did not plan for the loss of other friends. Typically, it is 11 year-old girls who pull worst-case shenanigans as described above. Do double milestoners mimic pre-adolescents? Sometimes.

In a best-case scenario, our mutual friends do not take sides.

However, even in these cases, it is reasonable to expect friendship fallout. For instance, tension mounts when current friends plan activities and decide to invite both our non-friend and us. What to do, especially if it is an anticipated special celebratory occasion? Do we attend knowing our ex-friend will be present, or refuse to attend and deprive ourselves of fun?

FOOD FOR THOUGHT

Give yourself the option to make decisions based on individual circumstances.

In an ordinary scenario, when friendships end, we are uncertain how to act toward each other in our new non-friend status. Depending on where we live, work, and socialize, we may encounter our former friends at social occasions, work functions, or shopping malls. Initially, it is natural to feel awkward. Fortunately, this discomfort is temporary and gradually tapers off after the first couple of meetings.

We cannot predict our ex-friend's reaction. What she does is up to her. (The same holds true for all our friends, including those who side with her and against us.)

Avoid becoming enemies – except in extreme circumstances. All we can control is our behavior. Even if it proves difficult, when seeing a former friend, be courteous and civil. A quick 'hello' is enough. Or, opt for a head nod.

HELPFUL HINT

Recently, I have developed a fondness for the simple head nod. It is a handy, often overlooked, gesture. Currently, mine are clumsy and silly. It is fun to sample different nods until finding one that becomes a *signature* nod.

MY STORY #1

I value honesty and do *not* lie. I do *not* attempt lying. This is a good strategy because I'm an awful liar. When seeing a former friend, I say, 'hello' but do *not* linger. I do *not* even say, 'how are you' because I do *not* want to engage in conversation. I do *not* say, 'it is good to see you.' Frankly, it is *not*. Told you I keep it honest (note the emphasis on all the '*I do nots*').

If my former friend initiates a conversation, I am polite and cordial, but avoid any attempts to rehash old stuff. Been there, done that. I do my best to make a graceful exit.

FOOD FOR THOUGHT

There is no need to be rude, disrespectful, or cruel to former friends. Lying and being phony is rude, disrespectful, and cruel – in my opinion.

MY STORY #2

When I assessed my friends according to the obnoxious cast of characters showcased in Chapter 6, it was evident I had a penchant for *attracting* Opera Singers. As already mentioned, in my pre-Swamp Goddess days, I was particularly drawn to One-Way Juanitas.

Typical Juanitas are expert at take, take, taking, while giving back mostly zilch, zero, nada. Harsh description – perhaps, accurate assessment – totally.

My completed SGFA Portions 1 & 2 revealed a few Keeper friends. I was relieved and happy. I acknowledged their unpleasant traits with humble recognition of my own. Overall, I decided these friends' desirable traits outweighed their undesirable ones. Hopefully, they felt the same when weighing my desirables and undesirables.

On the other hand, it was blatantly clear some friendships belonged on the Dump List. I was done making excuses for their Juanita personalities and giving two, three and, in some cases, forty-two chances. Thankfully, my Swamp Goddess self was finished with that. It was a no-brainer to end these friendships.

By now, we know Opera Singers do not pay close attention to others, except for how they are affected. My Swamp Goddess transformation managed to get my friends' attention. They actually noticed I changed the rules of our friendships.

I did not respond to my Opera Singer friends, nor was I available, in the ways I used to be. I began to ask for, and expect, certain friend *stuff* – reciprocity, mutual respect, and selfless acts of kindness. How dare I do this to Opera Singers, particularly One-Way Juanitas.

I am happy to report one Juanita friend changed as I

changed. She became a Keeper. Other Juanitas were not interested in me as Swamp Goddess. In fact, a couple ditched me before I could ditch them. More cheery news – they are not at all missed.

FOOD FOR THOUGHT

Turn about is fair play. Getting dumped works both ways. Do not be stunned if a friend says 'goodbye.' Based on her particular brand of menopausal mayhem and aging angst, a friend may conclude our behavior is unacceptable and let us go. Wicked!

Expect emotions to surface after friendships end, ranging from relief and exhilaration to sorrow and anger. Ideally, the good feelings will last; the bad will be transient.

Holding on to negative emotions is unhealthy. Yet, sometimes we are unable to fully release them. If you have tugged and pulled, but these feelings are hanging on, give yourself the gift of counseling.

A well-trained, reputable counselor will guide you through the process of assigning negative emotions a place of rest in your life story. She will dispense objective observations as you plan a course of action.

Letting go does not mean erasing the past. If only! Instead, we grasp that the past cannot be re-done. Plus, we learn how to prevent long ago events from defining or shaping our present and future. This is essential.

CHAPTER 11

I DO NOT KNOW WHAT TO DO WITH YOU

DESCRIPTION
After completing the Swamp Goddess Friendship Assessment, do you have friends who fit into The Unsure category? They have undesirable personality traits that are incompatible with your evolving Swamp Goddess self. In spite of this, you are reluctant to end the relationships. You believe (or want to believe) these friendships have potential … maybe … hopefully … please.

The following options will help clarify a plan for your Unsure friendships.

DIRECTIONS
Use pen and paper to record your responses.

⚙ To achieve the best outcome, complete The Swamp Goddess Friendship Assessment Portions 1 & 2.

- List the friends who fit The Unsure category.

- For each friend on the list, detail reasons why you are unsure.

Include

a) the desirable traits that foster your optimism for the future of this friendship.

b) the undesirable traits that foster your pessimism for the future of this friendship.

- Read the descriptions of the two options listed below.

- Choose the option that best suits each Unsure friendship.

a) OPTION #1 – The Friendship Break

b) OPTION #2 – The Big Talk

THE FRIENDSHIP BREAK
OPTION #1

DESCRIPTION
Stop all contact with your friend.

The Friendship Break is a cooling-off period or a trial separation. With a bit of physical and emotional distance, we gain a fresh perspective with which to decide if we want to continue or end a friendship.

How long does The Break last? It can be as long as you want.

The customary time frame is at least one month and at most six months.

Before you begin The Friendship Break agenda, you have to notify your friend. Sorry, you cannot simply disappear. Your friend will worry and wonder about your well-being. You may groan, 'I am not in the mood to inform her of anything.'

Question – Who is in the *mood* during the double milestone?
Answer – No one.

Question – What does it mean if you refuse to extend this courtesy?
Answer – It seems clear you have already decided to end the friendship.

If you are genuinely Unsure and there is a chance you can save the friendship, I advise writing a brief note telling your friend you're taking a Friendship Break. Assure her your health is fine. Do not explain or justify your actions. The less said (written), the better.

Just because you are evading a conversation, doesn't mean your friend feels the same. She may demand a face-to-face explanation. If you're not ready to see her or discuss your relationship, write that in the note.

The following is a sample note. It is best to be concise and aloof.

Hi Lulu:

I am writing to let you know I need to take a friendship break. Therefore, I will not be seeing or speaking to you for a while.

HELPFUL HINT

Note use of 'I' language. (See Chapter 12)

CAUTION!

It is almost impossible to accurately predict a friend's response to the cooling-off period. *You're* gambling she will accept *your* terms and be waiting when *you* decide The Break is over and *you* choose to resume the friendship. It is possible that when *you* designate *your* friend as a Keeper, she replies, 'too late' and tells *you* where to put *your* decisions. Are *you* willing to take this gamble?

MY STORY

After completing Portions 1 & 2 of The Swamp Goddess Friendship Assessment, I was left with a number of Unsure friendships. Were any of them were worth salvaging? I did not know.

I took The Friendship Break with a few Unsures. We had no contact. Depending on the friendship, The Break lasted between one and six months.

The cooling-off period exposed the emptiness of most of these friendships. They ended with scarcely a whimper. In retrospect, I realize each one of the Friendship Breaks served as a rehearsal for the actual breakups.

Also, The Friendship Break provided space for me to progress more fully into Swamp Goddess. Thereafter, decisions concerning my friends came easier and easier.

FOOD FOR THOUGHT

The Friendship Break is useful when the thought of having The Big Talk is too overwhelming. It is also a good choice if you have reached the two-friend limit reserved for The Big Talk.

CHAPTER 12

THE BIG TALK
OPTION #2

DESCRIPTION

Have you felt the need to tell your friend exactly how you feel? It is The Big Talk and it is A Big Deal. Reserve this for no more than one or two friends who fall into The Unsure category.

Selecting someone for The Big Talk requires earnest deliberation. Consider your friend's ability to engage in this type of discussion. You may be impatient to spill all, but your friend may not be ready, willing, and able to listen. Are you ready, willing, and able to listen to your friend's comeback? Really?

CAUTION!

- It is too draining to have The Big Talk with more than two friends (three if you must, but you'll be miserable).

- Never, ever, have The Big Talk with both friends at once. This will be disastrous.

FOOD FOR THOUGHT

It is crucial to be aware of your intentions and expectations.

BIG TALK INTENTIONS

The primary intention of The Big Talk is to facilitate the decision to keep or end a friendship. Other intentions have a tendency to slip in. These come in two flavors – positive or negative.

POSITIVE INTENTIONS

❂ Our aim is to give the friendship a chance to survive.

❂ We present changes we want and need.

❂ We offer realistic, fair, and doable proposals to enable the friendship to flourish.

NEGATIVE INTENTIONS

❂ Our aim is to confront our friend.

❂ We present evidence blaming her for everything wrong with the friendship.

❂ We do not propose any way for the friendship to continue.

❂ The plan is to express anger in such a way that she 'feels our pain.'

HELPFUL HINTS

I strongly urge using The Big Talk only if your intentions

are positive. If you have negative intentions, I encourage you to reconsider your plans. It is so very tempting to unleash a torrent of built-up disappointment, criticism, and rage at your soon-to-be ex friend. This type of encounter never has a good ending.

I am not suggesting stifling feelings or pretending things are all all right when they are not. If you know the friendship is finished, there is an alternative to the in-person confrontation.

An effective way to express disappointment, criticism, and rage is to write down what you want to say. Include the following.

DIRECTIONS
Use pen and paper to record your responses.

✿ Write down what you want to say to your friend.

✿ Organize all you have written into a letter.

✿ Once the letter is complete, put it in a drawer.

✿ In one week, read the letter out-loud to a photo of your friend.

✿ Optional – follow-up by engaging her in an imaginary dialogue.

✿ If needed, add and delete words, revise sentences, or rewrite the entire letter.

✿ When the letter accurately conveys your feelings, put it

back in the drawer.

✪ Reread the letter after two weeks and again after one month.

✪ Then, if you want to mail the letter to your friend, do so.

FOOD FOR THOUGHT

With time, the itch to send the letter usually passes and you are able to move on. If not, and you still want to send it, go to the local post office, buy a stamp, and mail your letter the old fashioned way. Sending and receiving a letter through the mail makes more of an impact than sending and receiving an email, text, or fax.

BIG TALK EXPECTATIONS

✪ Visualize the scene of The Big Talk.

✪ Imagine your friend's reaction.

✪ Be ready for a description of *your* imperfections. Yes, your friend gets a turn.

✪ Describe the potential aftermath of The Big Talk. What happens immediately afterward?

✪ What do you anticipate the long-term results to be?

DIRECTIONS FOR THE BIG TALK
Use pen and paper to record your responses.

✪ List your goals for The Big Talk.

❀ Write down everything you want to say.

❀ Call, text, or email your friend with an invitation to get together. Relay enough information so that she does not feel ambushed by your topic, but do not go into detail. It is best to wait for the in-person meeting.

❀ Although arrangements may be made by phone, text, or email, it is inadvisable to conduct The Big Talk by phone or email – and never by text or fax. If it is a long distance relationship, The Big Talk phone call is an option of last resort.

❀ Arrange uninterrupted time together. Keep both schedules free for approximately three hours. The discussion may take one hour or five minutes. Having extra time is handy, in case we need or want it.

BIG TALK PREPARATION

❀ The Big Talk should not be done spontaneously. It will dissolve into The Big Mistake. Careful planning and preparation are required.

❀ Do not let intrusions disrupt the event. Shut off all phones and other electronic devices. Some of us are very attached to our high-tech toys and cannot bear a separation. For this, you have to put them aside.

❀ Remember to bring reading glasses. Don't you hate assuming you're prepared, but those pesky glasses go missing and, without them, your notes are unreadable? Aaargh!

❀ Meet in a neutral spot, preferably where neighbors and

acquaintances will not stop to chat. Cafés, restaurants, or parks are fitting locations. Do not hold The Big Talk in either of your homes. It is not neutral, thereby giving an unfair edge to one of you.

☺ If you hold The Big Talk in a restaurant, stay away from alcohol. It clouds our heads and distorts our judgment. It is best to keep clear and focused. (That is, clear and focused in a double milestone sort of way.) Depending on the outcome of The Big Talk, have a drink afterward, toasting renewed friendship or mourning its end. Better yet, skip the alcohol and choose a delicious dessert. Yummy.

ADDITIONAL BIG TALK PREPARATION

☺ Organize your thoughts. Start with the most important point. Your friend may not stay to hear the rest. Her surprise may be that she turns your Big Talk into Short Talk.

☺ Practice using 'I' language (see Communication Tips).

☺ Avoid using 'You' language (see Communication Tips).

THE BIG TALK

☺ Present your thoughts clearly and briefly.

☺ Resist the very appealing urge to ramble, rant, or go off on tangents.

☺ Use one or two recent episodes to illustrate key concepts. Do not rehash events from last century.

☺ Exclude sweeping generalizations, such as 'never' and

'always.' For instance, 'you never call me' 'you always dominate conversations' are examples of unsuccessful communication techniques. Besides using provocative 'you' language, certainly there is at least one contradiction to those generalizations. Your friend can refute your claim by mentioning an exception, 'what about that time in 1972 when I called you.'

❀ Curb the temptation to recite a laundry list of grievances. It is overkill.

❀ Refrain from apologizing for stating your needs.

❀ Do not get defensive.

❀ Make no attempt to convince your friend of your sterling character. It is tempting, but unproductive.

THE GRAND FINALE

❀ Supply a proposal to save the friendship.

❀ Be explicit. What do you want? What do you need? If your plan is not to save the friendship, once again question your intentions and determine why you are having The Big Talk?

❀ When you finish your prepared speech, just stop. This step requires plenty of self-control. Easier said than done.

❀ The ball is now in your friend's court, so to speak. Her response is The Great Unknown.

ARE YOU EXHAUSTED YET?

FOOD FOR THOUGHT

All these steps accentuate the intensity of The Big Talk. Also, they underscore why it is essential to limit The Big Talk to one or two friends.

POTENTIAL RESPONSES

Your friend may react in one of the following ways.

1. She may

   ❂ listen carefully and hear your point of view.

   ❂ apologize.

   ❂ agree to your plan.

Or, let's get real.

2. She may

   ❂ refuse to listen.

   ❂ interrupt before your second sentence is spoken.

   ❂ get angry and lash out with her own grievances.

   ❂ weep and wail.

   ❂ walk out.

REMINDER

Be prepared for a wide variety of potential reactions.

CONNIE'S STORY

Connie was in distress because of her mother's serious illness. Her friend Julie did not offer any compassion. Moreover, Julie's aloof, detached actions disappointed Connie.

During Julie and Connie's Big Talk, it was Julie's pain that poured out. All of Julie's friends, including Connie, knew Julie was 14 when her own mother died. But, no one was aware that Julie's lingering, unresolved grief surfaced with the impending death of Connie's mom.

Grief, such as Julie's, leaves a residue of deep scars. During The Big Talk, Connie became fully aware of Julie's anguish.

FRIENDSHIP STATUS

The Big Talk revitalized Connie and Julie's friendship. Also Connie learned a powerful lesson. It is virtually impossible for one person to meet all our needs. In other words, stop expecting this impossibility.

Although Julie was unable to provide comfort for this matter, Connie was keenly aware of Julie's wonderful character. The friendship was indeed worth keeping.

In an unforeseen turn of events, Connie apologized to Julie for being insensitive. Connie admitted she was so absorbed in her grief, she was not mindful of Julie's history. Connie and Julie secured their friendship during a healing sob fest, topped off with soothing ice cream sundaes.

FOOD FOR THOUGHT

Connie's story is a sobering paradigm. We cannot assume, nor know everything. Connie was mistaking Julie's pain for lack of concern. She had it all wrong.

EMILY'S STORY

Emily was in a pitiful situation. She endured Alice's intolerable traits because Emily feared the *iffy* repercussions of having The Big Talk. Emily worried *if* she aired her complaints, Alice would end the friendship.

Emily had two friends. She was petrified *if* she lost Alice, just one friend would remain. What *if* the other friendship dissolved? Emily had a terrifying image of being elderly and friendless, with merely a small dog for company. She envisioned wandering the streets, pushing her furry pal in a doggie stroller. (Have you seen these?)

FRIENDSHIP STATUS
As of now, Emily chooses not to risk The Big Talk.

FOOD FOR THOUGHT

The Big Talk is iffy. On the other hand, settling for a problematic, unsatisfying friendship rather than risk being alone is dismal. The best choice for Emily is to widen her circle of friends (see chapter 13).

COMMUNICATION TIPS
'I' AND 'YOU' LANGUAGE

'I' LANGUAGE
We voice dissatisfaction (or satisfaction) to another person by articulating *our* personal perspective.

'YOU' LANGUAGE
We voice dissatisfaction to another person by pointing out *her* faults and mistakes.

EXAMPLES OF 'I' LANGUAGE
'I' language to a One-Way Juanita
'*I* want a reciprocal relationship balanced between give-and-take. *I* want my words heard and my feelings considered.'
'I' language version of Connie's Big Talk
'For the last month, *I* have attempted to discuss my mother's illness. *I* have cried and expressed my sorrow. *I* need to be listened to and consoled. *I* do not feel *I've* been getting what *I* need.'

HELPFUL HINT

These examples demonstrate speakers clearly stating their cases, without placing blame.

FOOD FOR THOUGHT

At first, 'I' language seems over-the-top and rather awkward. It takes a while before we get comfortable with this communication technique.

It is imperative to distinguish between 'I' language used in The Big Talk and 'I, I, I, Me, Me, Me' language of The Opera Singer Family. They are completely different.

'I' language expresses our thoughts and opinions relevant to specific discussions. The goal is to have fruitful dialogue and successful resolution. Others are present to be active participants.

For Opera Singers, all discussions revolve around them. Their goal is to orchestrate a monologue. Others are present to be receptacles.

'YOU' LANGUAGE

The effect of using 'you' language is often toxic. Most likely, the person with whom we are speaking hears it as hurling accusations, placing blame, and being attacked. She responds by becoming defensive and angry. Before we know it, the planned conversation gets out of hand and dissolves into a big mess.

EXAMPLES OF 'YOU' LANGUAGE
'You' language to a One-Way Juanita
'*You* are selfish, self-centered, and unreliable.' *You* call at all hours and *you* expect me to drop everything to serve *your* needs.'
'You' language version from Connie's Big Talk
'*You* are a bad friend. *You* do not offer comfort when I talk about my mom. *You* are cold and distant.'

HELPFUL HINT

These examples demonstrate speakers abrasively stating their cases by placing blame.

FOOD FOR THOUGHT

To have a productive outcome, I strongly advise against 'you' language, especially during The Big Talk. Ironically, 'you' language seems to come naturally and we need to suppress the inclination to use it.

HELPFUL HINT

Communication is a fascinating topic. Many instructive resources are available to sharpen our skills.

CHAPTER 13

SWAMP GODDESSES ON THE MOVE

As double milestoners move forward, we wonder whether it is possible to find new BFFs (Best Friends Forever) while navigating The Swamp Goddess path. Do you get nostalgic hearing teenagers use the phrase BFF? I do. It reminds me of my young, optimistic self when I believed in forever.

Because we have lived more than half of a century (isn't it alarming to see that in print), many of us are jaded by too many disappointments. Thus, BFFs, everlasting love, or anything promising our feelings will remain eternal, leave us with high levels of skepticism. Consequently, some of us are reluctant to let new people into our lives.

Additionally, as we age, opportunities to create relationships seem to be fewer. If there are chances to form new friendships, we notice they are slower to develop. Apparently, at the double milestone, we are not as flexible as we were at ten years old.

Not only can't we bend, run, and jump as nimbly as we did at ten, but our flexibility in other aspects of life has diminished as well – particularly opening ourselves to new people and experiences. Sheesh. Another flabby muscle, the friendship muscle.

Are we giving up? No, absolutely not. Double milestoners need to be creative in our quest to make friends. We do this by crafting a plan that uses our Swamp Goddess wisdom to find and develop quality friendships.

FOOD FOR THOUGHT

Aim for balance between caution and trust. It is reasonable to be cautious. Try to moderate caution by trusting yourself to make wise decisions.

REMINDER

You have completed The Swamp Goddess Friendship Assessment and know what you want and do not want. Be confident.

MORE FOOD FOR THOUGHT

Why not set different goals? For example

- ✪ *To have at least one BFFN (Best Friend For Now)*

- ✪ *To have at least one BBFN (Best Buddy For Now)*

WHERE DO SWAMP GODDESSES FIND NEW FRIENDS, BFFNS AND BBFNs?

❂ Focus on Quality not Quantity

Are you are sharing the ecstasy (just joking) of meno-pausal mayhem and aging angst with one or two fan-tastic friends? Consider yourself fortunate. If you have more, lucky you.

❂ Choose Friends from Desirable Families

Seek out Wise Wonderful Women, Gracious Glorious Gals, Fun Fab Femmes, Kind Caring Crew, Legendary Lovely Ladies, and House of Honorable Dames.

One friend from these desirable families is immeasura-bly superior to a dozen from undesirable ones.

❂ Busy, Busy, Busy

Keep active and participate in a variety of activities. The advice for finding a friend is identical to advice for find-ing a mate. It is based on the law of probability. That is, increased number of people you encounter=expanded selection=improved potential of meeting someone special.

❂ Widen The Circle

Push out of your comfort zone. To find quality friends, broaden your universe of possibilities to encompass people of various ages, ethnicities, and socioeconomic backgrounds. By the way, men make great friends.

✪ Differentiate Between Friends and Buddies

Success with this suggestion is more attainable after you complete The Swamp Goddess Friendship Assessment Portions 1 & 2. You will establish personal Friendship Criteria and acquire skills to effectively identify the differences between potential new friends and potential new buddies.

HELPFUL HINTS

✪ Friend = an individual who matches your Swamp Goddess Friendship Criteria.

✪ Buddy = an individual who does not match your Swamp Goddess Friendship Criteria, but you enjoy each other's company and share one or two common interests.

In pre-Swamp Goddess days (especially before completing The SGFA), many of us worked hard attempting to shape a *buddy* into a *friend.* We were continuously frustrated because we did not, could not, or would not accept that this aspiration was unachievable. Thanks to The SGFA, now we have tools to recognize a buddy relationship for what it is. We don't waste our efforts trying to make it what it's not, and never will be.

For example, you're introduced to somebody who is pleasant and fun. You both like watching horror movies and going gallery hopping. However, based on The Friendship Criteria you established, it is clear this person does not match your standards for a quality friendship. On the other hand, she does fit the description of buddy.

There is no reason for disappointment. Enjoy where and when your interests intersect without seeking more.

In other words, some involvements work perfectly as buddies, but not as friends, because the individual cannot – or will not – fit our Friendship Criteria. When we are clear on this and stop waiting for what we'll never get, our expectations change and our frustration is averted.

Adhering to your newly established Friendship Criteria demonstrates you'll no longer settle for less than what you want. Bravo! Swamp Goddesses do not settle.

FOOD FOR THOUGHT

We can enjoy activities with buddies. As long as we stay cognizant of the limitations, buddy relationships are amazingly liberating.

NOTE

Designating someone new in your life to buddy status is fairly effortless. Conversely, converting a current friend to buddy status is a challenging task.

It is comparable to the 'let's be friends' send-off we have all spoken, or heard, when ending a romantic relationship. Successfully shifting status remains an elusive outcome for most relationships – friendship, romantic, or otherwise.

SWAMP GODDESSES REACH OUT

In our search to develop quality friendships, many double milestoners are going back in time. Now, more than ever, we have the ability to reach out and transform old friends into midlife friends. Ideally, we seamlessly reprise at least one long-ago relationship.

In the past, every decade or so, we attended school reunions. It was fun to see childhood friends, update each other on our news, and walk down memory lane. Despite promises to keep in touch, most often we lost contact until the next reunion.

Social media has changed the way friends reconnect. Geography, work schedules, family obligations, and ... er ... weight gain, do not interfere with creating connections.

Online contact allows us many intriguing choices. We decide the types of reconnection we want and with whom, if – or when – to interact, and the limits we want to impose.

Do not be surprised if a few childhood friends are unresponsive to your rekindling overtures. For reasons we may never know, some folks are not receptive to recapturing the past and building a future with old friends. Don't take it personally. Just move forward.

FOOD FOR THOUGHT

It is worthwhile to double-check your expectations. Distinguish between fantasy and reality to keep those expecta-

tions grounded.

MORE FOOD FOR THOUGHT

Most importantly, turn the quest for new friends, BFFNs, and BBFNs into a fun, carefree adventure.

CHAPTER 14

FUTURE OLD FRIENDS

Can you envision your friendships at 85, 90, 95?

My mother and her group of friends may provide a peek into our futures. These women are in their mid to late 80s. While everyone's exact age is oddly private and closely guarded, mom and I delight in guessing how old each one is.

All the women are widowed and live alone. Assorted combinations of the larger group gather together in smaller clusters several times a week to play Mah Jong. It is a table game, fondly referred to as 'The Game.' Mah Jong resembles gin rummy. Rather than cards, tiles are used.

The women not only love Mah Jong, they need Mah Jong. The Game gives structure to their days, supplies treasured camaraderie, and provides respite from what would otherwise be virtual isolation.

Mom's group follows certain rituals and performs regular tasks for the Mah Jong Games. They deliberate over who will host upcoming Games, what snacks to serve, which Mah Jong rules to follow, and the ones to bend.

Every so often, The Game gets heated. I have observed arguing, cursing, and exchanging of angry outbursts. Mostly, it is because the women get agitated when a player spoils the fast-paced flow of Mah Jong by being too slow or making mistakes.

An impending eruption begins with telltale signs. One player impatiently drums her manicured fingernails on the table. Two other players alternate between tsk-tsking and loud sighing. The fifth player serves herself another piece of cake.

Usually, the bickering gets left at The Game table and is forgotten by the time the Mah Jong players go out for dinner.

There are instances when disagreements escalate into arguments. If peace is not swiftly restored, the situation can spiral downward. During the lull before the next Game, the telephone wires crackle with each group member giving her opinion, choosing sides, and adding to the drama.

Rifts may take weeks to heal. They eventually do, only to be replaced by new dramas. A couple of incidents have led to irreconcilable feuds. As a result, a few people have been ousted from The Game, and almost always, the group.

BACK TO THE FUTURE

I can't help but wonder if women time-travel as we enter our golden years? If so, this explains why my mother and her friends seem to have reverted to behavior typical of teenagers.

The older women exhibit adolescent-like behavior in the ways they rely on the group for companionship, support, and entertainment. The manner in which these elders relate to friends resembles teenage group behavior. They form cliques, gossip about – and argue with – each other, magnify minutiae to preposterous levels, and even use one another for personal gain.

Disputes eerily revive adolescent themes. A common one centers on feeling left out of the group. Remember the high school *in-crowd*? Who wants to revisit that popularity contest at 85?

THE IN-CROWD

Feelings get hurt when mom and her friends go to the local restaurant for their post Mah Jong meal. Because one dinner is too much food for each woman to eat by herself, two of them share one *early-bird special.* Problem: Five participants play Mah Jong, an uneven number.

Inevitably, somebody is left without a partner to share dinner. This woman may accept her fate, order a full dinner, and gracefully take home the leftover portion. Or, she may pout (sullen teenage posture and all) and refuse to order or eat anything.

FOOD FOR THOUGHT

It goes without saying, generally speaking, teenagers do not go to diners for early-bird specials. The key comparison between adolescents and these older women is the despair at being left out of their group. No matter our age, it is always painful when we are not chosen.

THE CAR

Another cause of disputes for mom's friends, reminiscent of teen behavior, is car related. Specifically, *can I get a ride?* And, *who sits up front?* Most in mom's age group no longer drive. In fact, many women of this generation never learned to drive or actually owned a car.

Among the Mah Jong players, one person has special power that comes from owning a car. She drives the women to The Game, the diner, and finally, their homes. Everyone wants to be her friend. More to the point, everyone wants to be her best friend. Not only to get a ride, but also to sit up front. Jostling for the ride and scrambling to get the status-seat is adolescence personified.

One of my mother's friends resides outside the driver's designated five-block driving radius and has to arrange her own transportation. This woman is shrewdly solving her plight by befriending a neighbor solely because she owns and drives a car.

Mom's friend constantly pesters the Mah Jong group to accept her car-driving neighbor into The Game. She aggressively promotes the advantages of having a back-up driver. No one likes the newcomer. Worse than that, she is a lousy player.

My mother predicts her friends will soon relent and allow the neighbor (and her coveted car) to join The Game, and eventually, the group.

SEXY SENIORS

For adolescents and elders, their generations' values influence their sexual attitudes and behaviors.

Are you astonished to learn that sexuality, specifically both generations' conversations pertaining to sex, are incongruously alike? Similar to teenagers, my mother's friends discuss sexual issues with a mixture of curiosity, awkwardness, and shyness. The two groups make silly wisecracks to cover their discomfort.

Each of my mother's friends is widowed to the man she married when very young. Supposedly, none dated after widowhood.

One day, my mother gleefully told me outrageous, game-stopping news (well ... almost). Mom and her friends found out that a member of the group is secretly dating men she meets through newspaper personal ads.

The women were barely recovered from that revelation, when even bigger news was divulged. Their friend is sexually active with her dates. This continues to be a sizzling hot topic.

FOOD FOR THOUGHT

Despite their petty spats and misunderstandings, these elderly women shine with the power of friendships. It's comforting to peek into the future and anticipate our Swamp Goddess golden years with cherished loved ones and close friends.

NOTE

I am delighted to share stories of my mother and her friends. This chapter was written when mom was alive. Sadly, she passed away and is missed so very much.

CHAPTER 15

FINAL WORDS

Thank you for taking The Swamp Goddess journey with me. We have shed light on the friendship frenzy that, for most of us, goes hand-in-hand with menopausal mayhem and aging angst.

Viewing friends through the specially-designed lens, The Swamp Goddess Friendship Assessment, is a bold accomplishment.

You have acquired techniques to

⚙ choose which friends to keep, those to let go, and know the difference.

⚙ create quality friendships that fit perfectly into your new Swamp Goddess lifestyle.

Congratulations.

FOOD FOR THOUGHT

If you have not yet completed SGFA portion 2, turn the page and get to it. The knowledge, insight, and skills you gain will strengthen your ability to make informed friend-ship choices.

MY STORY

When I began my Swamp Goddess journey, I asked myself the following double milestone questions.

✪ Where am I going?

✪ What am I going to do when I get there?

✪ Whom am I going with?

Any ideas? I still do not have the final answers to two of the questions. In response to the third one, I happily report that a couple of quality friends will be with me. I want the same for you. Mostly, I want all of us to have excellent Swamp Goddess stories. Ecstatic wishes!

THE BONUS ROUND

SWAMP GODDESS FRIENDSHIP ASSESSMENT (SGFA) PORTION 2

DESCRIPTION

There's no need for test anxiety or all night study sessions. Although I am a professor, The Swamp Goddess Friendship Assessment is not an exam. It is a learning tool.

The SGFA Portion 2 provides ample opportunities to effectively identify, assess, and change patterns of friendship-related behavior.

Specifically, you will
❀ pinpoint what you want and do not want.

❀ establish criteria.

❀ evaluate current friendships.

As an added benefit, you will
❀ acquire techniques to create quality friendships.

FOOD FOR THOUGHT

Here's an easy question to get The SGFA Portion 2 started.

Is it time to have the friendships you want, let go of those you don't, and know the difference?

Answer – Definitely!

DIRECTIONS
Use paper and pen to record your responses.

Portion 2 of The Swamp Goddess Friendship Assessment (SGFA) contains five sections.

- ✪ Carve out uninterrupted time. You may choose to do one section per day, one per week, or all 5 sections at once.

- ✪ As you begin each new section, do an initial read-through to familiarize yourself with its theme.

- ✪ Complete each section before you proceed to the next. The questions and the sections build on each other.

- ✪ Rather than formulating answers in your mind, write down your responses. Writing enhances the thought process. It also serves as a record for future review.

- ✪ Personalize the questions by tweaking them, if necessary, to suit you. Skip what does not apply.

CAUTION!

Do not trick yourself by skipping or ignoring difficult questions. Often, those are the consequential ones.

HELPFUL HINTS

For themes you deem especially meaningful, allow yourself extra time, but do not obsess. If you get stuck on a question, leave it and move on. Go back to that sticky question after the rest of that section is finished. Then, set a time limit and spend no more than one hour on that question.

FOOD FOR THOUGHT

Similar to THE SGFA Portion 1, Portion 2 may expose unresolved issues.

MORE FOOD FOR THOUGHT

The SGFA requires concentrated attention; something many of us haven't had since a few birthdays ago. The telltale signs of lost focus are quite familiar. We are distracted, thoughts wander, words vanish, and items mysteriously get misplaced.

Do you spend hours searching for that missing something – important document, crucial phone number, song title? This ridiculous searching takes up so much of my life, I now think of it as a part-time job.

Have you discovered a method to curtail roaming thoughts, retrieve meandering attention, and find lost items? Currently, I am on a quest for new remedies to shake off at least some of the accumulating brain fog and regain a modicum of focus. I test out an assortment of wholesome potentials.

Favorites include putting on music and dancing around my apartment. Sometimes (okay, many times), I get side-tracked, forget what I was originally looking for, and dance away into a new activity.

When this double milestone magic happens, I try my best to embrace it and *go with the flow*. Being upset at memory lapses, dwindling attention spans, and overall ditzy behavior is a dead end. Avoid dead ends. They lead nowhere.

SECTION 1

OBJECTIVE
Getting to know your friends

DIRECTIONS
Use pen and paper to record your responses.

☼ Retrieve your list of friends from SGFA Portion 1. This list will be used repeatedly.

☼ Next to every friend's name on your list, write down at least three qualities that describe her.

☼ Also, using your list of friends, answer the following:

- Name your oldest friend (length of time, not age).

- Name your closest friend.
  Why are you closest to her?

- Name the friend you like the best.

Why do you like her best?

- Name the friend you like the least.
Why do you like her least?

- How often do you see each friend?
Why this amount of time?

✪ Make note of any unexpected responses, insights, emotions, and thoughts.

FOOD FOR THOUGHT

'Why' questions and responses are extremely valuable. They foster awareness and insight by uncovering patterns and choices. 'Why' questions also provide opportunities to elaborate and expand thoughts and feelings.

SECTION 2

OBJECTIVE
To connect friends with our moods

DIRECTIONS
Use pen and paper to record your responses.

✪ From your list of friends, answer the following.

- Name the friend you prefer to be with when you are feeling happy. Why?

- Name the friend you evade when you are feeling happy. Why?

- Name the friend you turn to when you are feeling unhappy. Why?

- Name the friend you avoid when you are feeling unhappy. Why?

- Name the friend you consult when you need advice. Why?

- Do you consult the same friend for all types of advice? If Yes, name the friend.

- Do you consult different friends for different categories of advice, i.e. romance, family, career, fashion, health, other?

If your answer to a question is 'none,' provide explanations.

✪ Make note of any unexpected responses, insights, emotions, and thoughts.

REMINDER

More *why* questions lead to more valuable insights.

FOOD FOR THOUGHT

Have you begun to experience an array of emotions? There is no need to swallow them down or drown in the feelings. Just be aware they exist.

HELPFUL HINTS

At this point in The SGFA Portion 2, you may be racing to the end. Slow down. Tune into your reactions as you go through each step.

MORE HELPFUL HINTS

Is it time for a caffeine or food break yet? (I love an excuse to have chocolate.)

As an experiment, try taking an activity break. Fantastic news. For The SGFA only, walking to and from the fridge is considered physical activity. (We can add this to the wish list.)

If you are unable to resist floating into dreamland, snooze away. The SGFA will still be here when you awaken.

FOOD FOR THOUGHT

Naps are incredibly refreshing. They may be the only truly satisfying sleep we have during the double milestone.

SECTION 3

OBJECTIVE
To establish Friendship Criteria

DIRECTIONS
For the next set of questions, you need your list of friends and lots of paper.

Give each friend her own page.

PART A
To pinpoint Basic Personality Traits

DIRECTIONS
Use paper and pen to record your responses.

⚙ Read The Basic Personality Traits Scale.

⚙ Rate the 'level of importance' each Trait holds for you.

⚙ If it is 'important' your friends have a Trait, mark 'important.'

⚙ If it is 'unimportant' your friends have a Trait, mark 'unimportant.'

⚙ If it is 'somewhat important' your friends have a Trait, mark 'somewhat important.'

⚙ If you are 'unsure,' mark 'unsure.'

⚙ If you want to include additional traits, feel free to do so.

BASIC PERSONALITY TRAITS SCALE

Honest	Generous
Smart	Sense of humor
Fun	Responsible
Reliable	Optimistic
Loyal	Polite
Supportive	Assertive
Happy	Honorable
Trustworthy	Spontaneous
Wise	Calm

Independent	Kind
Intelligent	Thoughtful
Easy Going	Introspective
Well Groomed	

PART B
To review your responses

DIRECTIONS
Use paper and pen to record your responses. Refer to The Personality Traits Scale to answer the following.

❂ Write a list of The Basic Personality Traits you rated 'important.'

❂ Write a list of The Basic Personality Traits you rated 'unimportant.'

❂ Write a list of The Basic Personality Traits you rated 'somewhat important.'

❂ Write a list of The Basic Personality Traits you rated 'unsure.'

❂ Which list is the longest? Which list is the shortest?

❂ Write a description of your reactions.

❂ Make note of any unexpected responses, insights, emotions, and thoughts.

MORE QUESTIONS TO PONDER

❂ Do you have an unanticipated number of 'unsures?'

✪ Are you curious regarding your 'unsures' and wonder why you do not have definitive responses? Simple answer. Before now, you did not have access to The Swamp Goddess Friendship Assessment.

EXTRA CREDIT

✪ Refer to The Personality Traits you rated 'important.'

✪ Are you willing to be friends with someone who does not have The Personality Traits you rated 'important?'

✪ Be specific in detailing why or why not.

PART C
To assign scores

DIRECTIONS
Use paper and pen to record your responses. Refer to your original list of friends. Each friend will be assigned a score based on Basic Personality Traits.

✪ For every Basic Personality Trait you rated 'important,' write that Trait with a score of '3' next to each friend who *has* that Trait.

✪ For every Basic Personality Trait you rated 'important,' write that Trait with a score of '2' next to each friend who *somewhat has* that Trait.

✪ For every Basic Personality Trait you rated 'important,' write that Trait with a score of '1' next to each friend who *does not have* that Trait.

✪ If you are *unsure*, write that Trait and 'unsure' next to your friends' names.

HELPFUL HINTS

1=your friend *does not have* the Trait you rated 'important.'

2=your friend *somewhat has* the Trait you rated 'important.'

3=your friend *has* the Trait you rated 'important.'

MORE HELPFUL HINTS

For example, you rated 'honesty' as 'important.'

If your friend Ruby *is* 'honest,' she scores a '3.' She *has* the Trait 'honesty.'

On your list of friends, next to Ruby's name, write 'honesty=3.'

If your friend Joyce *is not* 'honest,' she scores a '1.' She *does not have* the Trait 'honesty.'

On your list of friends, next to Joyce's name, write 'honesty=1.'

PART D

To assess how your friends measure up

DIRECTIONS

Use paper and pen to record your responses.

⚙ Make separate categories for each of the following.

⚙ Record the friends who scored '3s.' They *have* Basic Personality Traits you rated 'important.'

⚙ Record the friends who scored '2s.' They *somewhat have* Basic Personality Traits you rated 'important.'

☢ Record the friends who scored '1s.' They *do not have* Basic Personality Traits you rated 'important.'

☢ Record the friends who scored 'unsures.' You are *unsure* if they have Basic Personality Traits you rated 'important.'

PRELIMINARY ASSESSMENT

☢ Has one friend scored '3s' on all Basic Personality Traits you rated 'important?' You are off to a great start. If two or more friends scored '3s,' give a big cheer. You are fortunate.

☢ Maybe, none of your friends scored '3s,' and your list of friends is filled with scores of '1s,' Sigh! I'll bet you have a whopper of a hot flash right about now. Take a few deep breaths, drink a glass of cold water, fan yourself, and keep going. Hopefully, the next two surveys will show better results.

☢ Perhaps, many friends scored '2s.' Ask yourself if you are settling for crumbs rather than the whole loaf. Hmmm ... something to think about.

☢ Keep track of 'unsures.' Specifically, what caused you to be 'unsure?'

FOOD FOR THOUGHT

Viewing friendships through The Swamp Goddess Lens magnifies our double milestone vision. We are able to 'see' what previously went unnoticed.

PART E
To pinpoint Common Ground Traits

DIRECTIONS
Use paper and pen to record your responses.

⚙ Read each Common Ground Trait listed below.

⚙ Rate the 'level of importance' each Common Ground Trait holds for you.

⚙ If it is 'important' your friends and you share a Common Ground Trait, mark 'important.'

⚙ If it is 'unimportant' your friends and you share a Common Ground Trait, mark 'unimportant.'

⚙ If it is 'somewhat important' your friends and you share a Common Ground Trait, mark 'somewhat important.'

⚙ If you are 'unsure,' mark 'unsure.'

⚙ If you want to include additional traits, feel free to do so.

COMMON GROUND SCALE

Similar schedule	Same religion
Similar education	Sameculture/ethnicity
Similar income level	Same marital status
Similar lifestyle	Same political ideology
Same neighborhood	Shared values
Same age	Shared history
Same race	Shared interests

Shared confidences   Shared time

EXTRA CREDIT

⊛ If you rated Shared Values as 'important,' what specific values are most 'important to share' with friends?

⊛ If you rated Shared Time as 'important,' how much time do you need to spend together to maintain a friendship?

⊛ If you rated Shared Interests as 'important,' what interests are most 'important to share' with friends?

⊛ If you rated Shared Confidences as 'important,' what topics, if any, would you *not* share, i.e. topics you consider off-limits and will not reveal?

⊛ What topics do you *not* want your friends to share with you, i.e. topics you consider off-limits and do not want your friends to reveal?

PART F
To review your responses

DIRECTIONS
Use paper and pen to record your responses. Refer to The Common Ground Scale to answer the following.

⊛ Write a list of Common Ground Traits you rated 'important.'

⊛ Write a list of Common Ground Traits you rated 'unimportant.'

❂ Write a list of Common Ground Traits you rated 'somewhat important.'

❂ Write a list of Common Ground Traits you rated 'unsure.'

❂ Which list is the longest? Which is the shortest?

❂ Write a description of your reactions.

❂ Make note of any unexpected responses, insights, emotions, and thoughts.

EXTRA EXTRA CREDIT

❂ Refer to The Common Ground Traits you rated 'important.'

❂ Are you willing to be friends with someone who does not share The Common Ground Traits you rated 'important?'

❂ Be specific in detailing why or why not.

FOOD FOR THOUGHT

Were there any surprises concerning The Common Ground Traits you rated 'important' and 'unimportant?' What about 'unsures?' Are you still questioning how it's possible to be 'unsure' of what is 'important?' The answer remains easy. Before now, you did not have access to The Swamp Goddess Friendship Assessment.

Part G
To assign scores

DIRECTIONS

Use paper and pen to record your responses. Refer to your list of friends. Each friend will be assigned a score based on Common Ground Traits.

❁ For every Common Ground Trait you rated 'important,' write that Trait with a score of '3' next to each friend with whom you *share* that Trait.

❁ For every Common Ground Trait you rated 'important,' write that Trait with a score of '2' next to each friend with whom you *somewhat share* that Trait.

❁ For every Common Ground Trait you rated 'important,' write that Trait with a score of '1' next to each friend with whom you *do not share* that Trait.

❁ If you are unsure, write that Trait and 'unsure' next to your friends' names.

HELPFUL HINTS
1=your friend *does not share* the Common Ground Trait you rated 'important.'

2=your friend *somewhat shares* the Common Ground Trait you rated 'important.'

3=your friend *shares* the Common Ground Trait you rated 'important.'

MORE HELPFUL HINTS
For example, you rated 'same political ideology' as 'important.'

If your friend Ruby and you *share* 'same political ideology,' she scores a '3.'

On your list of friends, next to Ruby's name, write 'political ideology=3.'

If you rated 'political ideology' as 'important,' but your friend Joyce and you *do not share* the 'same political ideology,' she scores a '1.'

On your list of friends, next to Joyce's name, write 'political ideology=1.'

PART H
To assess how your friends measure up.

DIRECTIONS
Use paper and pen to record your responses.

- ✪ Make separate categories for each of the following.

- ✪ Record the friends who scored '3s.' You *share* Common Ground Traits you rated 'important.'

- ✪ Record the friends who scored '2s.' You *somewhat share* Common Ground Traits you rated 'important.'

- ✪ Record the friends who scored '1s.' You *do not share* Common Ground Traits you rated 'important.'

- ✪ Record the friends who scored 'unsures.' You are *unsure* if they share Common Ground Traits you rated 'important.'

PRELIMINARY ASSESSMENT

❂ Has one friend scored '3s' on all Common Ground Traits you rated 'important?' Shout with delight. If two or more friends scored all '3s,' roar with gratitude.

PART I
To pinpoint your Tolerance Level. Who is getting on your last nerve?

DIRECTIONS
Use paper and pen to record your responses.

❂ Read each Bothersome Trait listed below.

❂ Rate your 'Tolerance Level' for each Bothersome Trait.

❂ If the Trait is 'intolerable,' mark 'intolerable.'

❂ If the Trait is 'somewhat tolerable,' mark 'somewhat tolerable.'

❂ If the Trait is 'tolerable,' mark 'tolerable.'

❂ If you are 'unsure,' mark 'unsure.'

❂ Feel free to add other Bothersome Traits that impact your Tolerance Level

THE TOLERANCE SCALE

Competitive	Angry
Jealous	Unhappy
Pessimistic	Controlling
Petty	Aggressive
Clingy	Gloomy

Self-absorbed	Perfectionist
Sloppy	Rude
Needy	Unkempt
Manipulative	Inconsiderate
Complainer	Selfish
Argumentative	Sad
Assertive	Dishonest
Untrustworthy	Greedy
Stingy	

PART J
To review your responses.

DIRECTIONS
Use paper and pen to record your responses. Refer to The Tolerance Scale to answer the following.

- ❂ Write a list of Bothersome Traits you rated 'intolerable.'

- ❂ Write a list of Bothersome Traits you rated 'tolerable.'

- ❂ Write a list of Bothersome Traits you rated 'somewhat tolerable.'

- ❂ Write a list of Bothersome Traits you rated 'unsure.'

- ❂ Which list is the longest? Which list is the shortest?

- ❂ Write a description of your reactions.

- ❂ Make note of any unexpected responses, insights, emotions, and thoughts.

EXTRA CREDIT

✪ Refer to The Bothersome Traits you rated 'intolerable.'

✪ Are you willing to be friends with someone who has The Bothersome Traits you rated 'intolerable?'

✪ Be specific in detailing why or why not.

FOOD FOR THOUGHT

Are you surprised at the Bothersome Traits you rated 'tolerable' and 'intolerable?' With age, our 'tolerance level' undergoes amazing changes and bewildering shifts. It can be confusing. How is it that circumstances we used to hardly notice, now really annoy us? In contrast, we are more 'tolerant' of stuff that used to be unbearably irritating.

Again, this is to be expected. Aging wisdom has altered our perspective. We are at a special time in life when certain things (and people) aggravate us, while others do not matter much anymore, especially when viewed through The Swamp Goddess Lens. Could it be more evidence of double milestone magic … or something?

PART K
To assign scores

DIRECTIONS
Use paper and pen to record your responses.

Refer to your original list of friends. Each friend will be assigned a score based on your Tolerance Level for Bothersome Traits.

❂ For every Tolerance Level Trait you rated 'intolerable,' write that Trait with a score of '3' next to each friend who *does not have* that Trait.

❂ For every Tolerance Level Trait you rated 'intolerable,' write that Trait with a score of '2' next to each friend who *somewhat has* that Trait.

❂ For every Tolerance Level Trait you rated 'intolerable,' write that Trait with a score of '1' next to each friend who *has* that Trait.

❂ If you are unsure, write that Trait and 'unsure' next to your friends' names.

HELPFUL HINTS
1=she *has* the 'intolerable' Trait.

2=she *somewhat has* the 'intolerable' Trait.

3=she *does not have* the 'intolerable' Trait.

MORE HELPFUL HINTS
For example, you rated 'manipulative' as 'intolerable.'

If your friend Ruby *is not* 'manipulative,' she scores a '3.' She *does not have* the Trait 'manipulative.'

On your list of friends, next to Ruby's name, write 'manipulative=3.'

If your friend Joyce *is* 'manipulative,' she scores a '1.' She *has* the Trait 'manipulative.'

On your lists of friends, next to Joyce's name, write

'manipulative=1.'

PART L
To assess how your friends measure up.

DIRECTIONS
Use paper and pen to record your responses.

⚙ Record the names of friends who scored '3s.' They *do not have* Bothersome Traits you rated 'intolerable.'

⚙ Record the names of friends who scored '2s.' They *somewhat have* Bothersome Traits you rated 'intolerable.'

⚙ Record the names of friends who scored '1s.' They *have* Bothersome Traits you rated 'intolerable.'

⚙ Record the friends who scored 'unsures.' You are *unsure* if they have Bothersome Traits you rated 'intolerable.'

PRELIMINARY ASSESSMENT

⚙ If you have one friend who does not have any Bothersome Traits, jump for joy.

⚙ How many of your friends have more than one Bothersome Trait? Do they all have the same Bothersome Trait? This is fairly common.

FOOD FOR THOUGHT

Contemplate why you have friends with Traits you consider 'intolerable.' Is there a trade-off? Sometimes, we tolerate the intolerable by convincing ourselves that, overall, a friend's desirable qualities outweigh her undesirable qualities. Are you sure?

NOT SO EASY EXTRA EXTRA CREDIT

☺ Test out the desirable/undesirable equation.

☺ Using the awareness and insights gathered from The SGFA, go back to your original list of friends.

☺ Next to each friend's name write yourself a letter explaining why you tolerale her intolerable traits.

☺ Determine if the trade-off is worth it. Decide what you are willing to accept.

☺ Yikes! Seeing this equation written out is a powerful reality check.

SECTION 4

OBJECTIVES
To establish Friendship Criteria.

To reveal your Keepers, Non Keepers (Dumpees), and Unsures.

DIRECTIONS
☺ Review the results elicited from all three: Basic Personality, Common Ground, and Tolerance Level Scales.

✪ Compile two new lists.

✪ One list is comprised of all Traits you rated 'important' on The Basic Personality and Common Ground Scales. This is your personal Friendship Criteria. Swamp Goddesses expect our friends to have Traits we rated 'important.'

✪ The second list is comprised of all Bothersome Traits you rated 'intolerable' on The Tolerance Level Scale. This is also part of your personal Friendship Criteria, specifically what you do *not* want. Swamp Goddesses are not willing to accept the 'intolerable.' Why should we?

RESULTS, PLEASE – NAMING NAMES

List your friends who scored '3s' on The Basic Personality, Common Ground, and Tolerance Level Scales. Has at least one friend scored '3s' on every scale? Very Impressive! Do you have two or more friends who scored '3s' on every scale? Stellar! Whether it is one or five friends who fit this category, celebrate your blessings. Tell each one how much you value the friendship.

If none of your friends scored '3s', Owww! There is a silver lining. Now that the results are out in the open, you know what needs to be changed and have the necessary tools to move forward.

List your friends who scored '1's on: The Basic Personality, Common Ground, and Tolerance Scales. If you have friends who fit this category, A Howling Owww! Don't you agree it is time to free yourself from them and make room for quality friendships?

List your friends who scored '2's on The Basic Personality, Common Ground, and Tolerance Scales. You have serious thinking to do regarding these friends.

SECTION 5

OBJECTIVE
To gain awareness of yourself as a friend. You may have heard the saying 'to have a friend, you have to be a friend.'

It is time to survey you. Your turn.

DIRECTIONS
Use paper and pen to record your responses.

You need your original list of friends.

⚙ Next to each name, detail what you contribute to sustain and nurture the friendship.

⚙ Do you *need* to make more of an effort? In what ways?

⚙ Do you *want* to make more of an effort? Why or why not?

FOOD FOR THOUGHT

All friendships require upkeep. Different friendships require different types of upkeep.

THE NEXT STEP

Take a breather. Allow yourself time to process the results of SGFA Portion 2. When you are ready to implement The SGFA, proceed to Chapter 9 and beyond.

Combine your newly acquired skills to a bit of fervent determination and you will be well-equipped to navigate the double milestone - ideally with a few quality friends alongside.

WHAT IS IT ALL ABOUT?

You have completed The Swamp Goddess Friendship Assessment. Well Done!

Now you have enhanced knowledge, insight, and skills to

✪ ease your passage through the murky waters of menopausal/aging friendship frenzy.

✪ choose which friends to keep, those to let go, and know the difference.

✪ create quality friendships that fit perfectly into your new Swamp Goddess lifestyle.

Plus, you no longer have to wonder, "Is it me? Am I the only menopausal/midlife woman chanting the silent roar, Help! I am surrounded by bitches ... oops, I mean friends?" Best wishes!

ACKNOWLEDGEMENTS

I am grateful to, and for, my family and friends. They are wonderful traveling companions on The Swamp Goddess journey.

My best friends are my terrific sisters, Marsha Wohl and Leslye Schottenfeld.

My amazing nephew Josh's encouragement propelled me past the final hurdle. My other nephews Brian, Todd, and Peter are amazing as well.

Marsha Wohl, Leslye Schottenfeld, Margie Polan Tellez, Suzanne Gulbin, and Cristine Levitre responded generously when called upon to be readers. I appreciate their valuable feedback and thoughtful comments. Louise Santamaria and Amy Beanland were kind enough to read parts of a preliminary draft and offered helpful suggestions.

Suzanne Gulbin expertly, reliably, and patiently guided me through the intricacies of social networking. Nancy Arum has been a cohort in Swamp Goddess dreams. Margie Telez reminds me there's magic in forever friendships. Russell

Young asked thought-provoking questions and coached useful responses. My author buddies are a talented, fun group willing to impart their know-how. I learn so much from them.

The women who shared their stories of friendship frenzy are the foundation of *Help! I Am Surrounded By Bitches…* I am thankful for their contributions.

Most of all, deep love, admiration, and appreciation go to my son, Jesse Scaturro. He was the first person with whom I shared the concept for this book. Jesse lit the spark that became The Swamp Goddess and created hilarious depictions of Opera Singers and their endless 'I, I, I, Me, Me, Me' rants.

Jesse's expert artistic contributions have been integral to this project. He designed a Swampy cover, filmed and directed the trailer, shot my author photograph, plus created an awesome web site and blog. Obviously, I have kept Jesse busy.

From that long ago discussion, through completion, Jesse has been my main source of wise counsel and trusted support. Thanks, Jess. I adore you.

ABOUT THE AUTHOR

As a college professor for 25 years, Wendy Kyman, Ph.D. has taught Women's Health, Human Sexuality, and Nutrition courses. As a therapist, she has conducted seminars and counseled women on a vast array of topics, including aging and menopause. These roles, plus Dr. Kyman's personal experiences, are instrumental in chronicling anecdotes of women's journey through menopause and midlife.

www.midlifememos.com

www.ingramcontent.com/pod-product-compliance
Lightning Source LLC
Chambersburg PA
CBHW050122280326
41933CB00010B/1212